Praise

"In *Saving Sam*, Jay Cohn, an eminent cardiovascular researcher and clinician, has chronicled his personal experience in understanding the causes and treatments of heart diseases, and has done so with great clarity and insight. This is a marvelous book that demonstrates how one physician-scientist has realized a goal few of us can ever hope to achieve— pursuing a research focus that ultimately directly benefits our patients."

Joseph Loscalzo, M.D., Ph.D.,
Chairman, Department of Medicine,
Brigham and Women's Hospital
Hersey Professor of the Theory and Practice of Medicine
Harvard Medical School

"*Saving Sam* is a remarkable medical adventure. Dr. Cohn makes the reader feel the excitement of new insights into disease mechanisms and the development of drugs to treat hypertension and heart failure. This is a remarkable journey through the beginnings of modern heart failure therapy to the future of heart failure and cardiovascular disease prevention with a master clinician, clinical investigator and teacher."

Bertram Pitt, M.D.
Professor of Medicine Emeritus, University of Michigan

In Saving Sam, Dr. Cohn clarifies many of the details about the BiDil controversy that I was not aware of at the time. It was difficult for me to really understand why the concept that not all patients respond similarly to therapy was so foreign to the critics. I'm sure the criticism he writes about was hurtful. Through the pure force of his intellect, Cohn was able to deal with much of the hostility.

Dr. Gary S. Francis
Professor of Medicine, University of Minnesota

"An exceptional depiction of the development of afterload moderating agents and their moderation of hypertension, heart failure, renal failure and, as we later learned, even erectile dysfunction. At the same time the book gives us a fascinating look at medical training in an era when understanding the history of a patient and a caring physician were the standard. This book is highly recommended."

Eric Sabety, M.D.

Orthopedic Surgeon

Saving Sam

Drugs, Race, and Discovering the Secrets of Heart Disease

Jay Cohn, MD

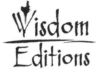

an imprint of
Calumet Editions, Minneapolis, Minnesota, USA

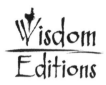

an imprint of
Calumet Editions, Minneapolis, Minnesota, USA

FIRST EDITION OCTOBER 2014

SAVING SAM: Drugs, Race, and Discovering
the Secrets of Heart Disease

For information regarding bulk purchases or author availability, please contact Calumet Editions at 952-937-0182, or e-mail us at
info@calumeteditions.com

Printed in the United States of America.

Library of congress Cataloguing-in-Publication Data
has been applied for.

ISBN – 9781939548122

10 9 8 7 6 5 4 3 2 1

Cover art and book design by Gary Lindberg

Saving Sam

Drugs, Race, and Discovering the Secrets of Heart Disease

Jay Cohn, MD

Acknowledgments

This book could not have been written without the tolerance and support of my wife, Syma Cheris Cohn, who has shared my life for more than 60 years and has inspired me with her poet's dedication to words and her art historian's dedication to form.

The ideas and discoveries recounted here were a product of experiences shared with a number of collaborators over the years. Many, but not all, are identified in the text for their contributions to specific experiences described. To those and others I extend my deep appreciation for their intellectual and physical contributions.

Much of the artwork included in the book was produced by Bill Dobbs, a graphic artist in Minneapolis. His skill in depicting the anatomical diagrams is greatly appreciated.

My publisher, Calumet Editions, has provided valuable advice in improving and targeting the text. Ian Graham Leask offered remarkable insight over many months of revisions and reorganization. Gary Lindberg was a superb advisor and editor in discarding unnecessary words and tightening the text. Their efforts have been critically important to the final product.

Finally, I must thank the many patients and colleagues who have stimulated the quest for knowledge that is reflected in this work.

Dedication

To the patients, their families, their care givers, and the basic and clinical scientists who have shared in my quest for a better understanding of these diseases and their management

TABLE OF CONTENTS

PREFACE

When William Harvey first described the circulation of blood in 1628, he had no idea of the complexity of the heart and attached network of blood vessels that we now call the cardiovascular system. Harvey, a physician, was passionate about the circulation and wanted to learn more. So did an artist, Leonardo da Vinci, who more than 100 years before Harvey had painstakingly drawn the details of the heart and blood vessels using human corpses as the model. Da Vinci had concluded that the system was designed to move blood out of the heart and into the network of arteries. Neither of these creative minds could have imagined what we have learned about this remarkable system, and that disturbances in it are the world's major cause of disability and death.

Harvey clarified that blood circulates through the arteries and veins propelled by the force of the heart's rhythmic contraction. During the subsequent 350 years, physicians and scientists focused on the heart, its rhythm, the nourishment of its working muscle, its pumping power, and its ability to provide adequate blood flow to the vital organs of the body. When patients became sick because of inadequate circulation, the heart's ability to pump blood drew the attention of care givers. Surgical techniques for correcting structural abnormalities of the heart became available in the 20th century, as did implanted electrical devices to resolve heart rhythm problems. But when heart muscle weakened, there was little that could be done. This was the situation I faced when completing my medical training in the early 1960s.

During the past 50 years the revolution in our understanding and treatment of the cardiovascular system has been breath-taking. Nonetheless, cardiovascular diseases—heart attacks, strokes, sudden death, heart failure, kidney failure, inadequate blood flow to the legs or brain—still disables or kills most of us. I am convinced that this need not be the case in the future. My commitment to unlocking the mysteries of cardiovascular disease and developing new ways to treat it began during my Boston internship in 1956 and continues to this day. My life has been dedicated to finding and using more effective therapies that can prevent disease from progressing and prolong life. The goal is to change the future for everyone in countries where an aging population increases the risk for cardiovascular disease.

This book is an effort to provide insights critical to understanding the common diseases that plague us. The media thrive on over-simplification. Diet, lifestyle and stress are often trumpeted as the villains. A particular behavior pattern or pill may be identified as the cause of heart attacks, or a means of protecting us from them. People who read these reports may become anxious about their personal risk. Patients have asked me if they should stop taking a medication suddenly found to be "risky", or if they should get a dog because pet ownership has been found to be associated with improved survival. Unfortunately, the media and the public often fail to understand the difference between *relative risk* and *absolute risk*. And the difference between an *observational study* and a *prospective study* seems to escape most of them.

A specific medication or life style may be reported as decreasing the risk of heart attack by 20%. That sounds like a big effect, but if the risk of a heart attack for an individual over 10 years is 1 in 20, then a 20% decrease would bring the risk to 0.8 in 20, a preciously small change. Observational studies, which compare two populations of people, do not account for baseline differences. People who own pets, for example, may have different characteristics or lifestyles from those who don't. The only way to really determine if, for example, pet ownership alters risk is to start with a population without a pet and randomly assign half to acquire a pet and the other half not. Studying the outcomes in these two groups is the gold standard of *prospective* clinical trials.

Cardiovascular disease is influenced by so many inherited and environmental factors that no single strategy can be advocated for everyone. We are all different. No recommendation is equally effective for all people. The public would like simple answers, but they don't exist. When it comes to medical treatment "one size" does not "fit all".

We are in an era when the medical profession demands evidence to support treatment strategies. New therapies get studied in thousands of patients to determine their effectiveness and their safety. Such studies are mandated by regulators such as the Food and Drug Administration (FDA), which controls the approval and marketing of new treatments for human diseases. These large trials are carried out in specific subpopulations that have those diseases. Selecting a "responsive" population is at the core of effective drug development. We all know that everyone does not respond in the same way.

Recognition of the variability of human responses has led to the current demand for personalized medicine. This concept was popularized after the human genome project made it possible to explore the entire genetic background of each individual, and theoretically to determine how every variation in the genome is translated into a disease and its response to a potential treatment. The naïve hope that personalized medicine based on genomic analysis was just "around the corner" has been dashed as we learned that few diseases, and little of the variability in their response to treatment, can be explained by single genetic variables or mutations. The complexity of using the genome to drive personalized medicine limits its practical use in clinical medicine today.

Is there an alternative to genomic "personalized medicine?"

The biological process that leads to heart attacks, strokes and other cardiovascular diseases occurs in the cardiovascular system—the heart and arteries studied by da Vinci and Harvey. Damage begins there, and progresses over many years into these morbid events. Abnormalities of the heart and arteries can be detected long before people experience symptoms and die. Measurable abnormalities of the heart and blood vessels vary immensely from patient to patient, and the degree of severity is the major determinant of whether symptomatic disease will occur.

For diagnostic purposes we lump people into disease categories that are largely arbitrary. When blood pressure is above a certain level the profession has decided to call it hypertension. When blood sugar is above a certain level we call it diabetes. When cholesterol exceeds some arbitrary threshold we give it a name and call it a disease. These are not necessarily diseases unless we choose to call them that. People rarely die because their blood pressure, blood sugar or cholesterol is too high. Our concern is that patients with numbers that are too high are at increased risk to die from cardiovascular disease. But that increased risk is related to whether they develop measurable abnormalities in the arteries or the heart.

Identifying the nature and severity of abnormalities of the heart and blood vessels, and monitoring the response of these abnormalities to treatment, potentially offer the personalized medicine not yet delivered by genomics. We know that genes play a key role in determining the nature and severity of these abnormalities and their responsiveness to treatment, but genomic analysis is still in its infancy. Fortunately, we have some substitutes for genomics, imperfect as they are. These may be considered "surrogates", or substitutes for the real culprit, the gene. Gender, geographic origin, ethnicity or race, body size, hair color, eye color are all determined in part by genes. In an effort to personalize medicine, no trait that is associated with disease can be ignored.

The quest to understand the structural and functional abnormalities associated with cardiovascular disease has been pursued by many investigators in the last half-century. My laboratory and colleagues—first in Washington, D.C., and then at the University of Minnesota—have been at the forefront of many conceptual advances during those years. Fundamental to many of these insights was the development of a better treatment for the failing heart that relied on a previously unrecognized property of the pumping heart. The discovery that a drug which relaxes the arteries could also improve the function of the heart became the first conceptual advance in the management of heart failure since the illness was first described. That discovery led to a new drug, BiDil, which has been the focus of intense controversy over the eight years since FDA approval.

On June 16, 2005 the Cardiorenal Advisory Committee of the FDA met at a Holiday Inn in Gaithersburg, Maryland, and unanimously recommended that BiDil, which I had invented by combining two generic drugs, be approved for treatment of heart failure in black patients. The event received widespread media coverage both before and after the meeting. The stock of the small public company that would market the drug soared.

Interest in this approval was intense for several reasons, the most obvious being that it would be the first drug approved for a single racial subgroup of the population. Although many sociologists, anthropologists and geneticists railed against this so-called racial profiling in medical therapy, the FDA made light of the complexity of such a decision. The clinical trial, A-HeFT, that served as the basis for the FDA approval was carried out exclusively in self-identified black African Americans, a strategy the FDA had recommended after examining our preliminary data. The trial demonstrated a 43% reduction in mortality in the patients given BiDil compared to those given a placebo. FDA guidelines state that approval of a drug and its marketing be limited to the population in whom the drug was proved effective. The FDA had no problem approving BiDil for black patients with heart failure.

Unfortunately, that simple and seemingly rational action turned out to be neither simple nor as rational as the FDA might have assumed. Some critics noted that studies performed in nearly all white populations lead to approval for everyone without reference to race. Why, they complained, should a study performed in blacks be approved only for blacks? They insisted that this was clearly a double standard: Whites represent "everyone"; blacks represent only blacks. The FDA defended its position by noting that in prior studies blacks were merely un-der-represented, whereas in this study non-blacks were excluded. No non-blacks were given the drug, they noted, so it couldn't yet be approved for whites or other racial groups.

The FDA's stance on drug approval is based on its recognition of the variability in human responses. If certain individuals are unresponsive to a specific drug, or have a high side effect risk from the drug, it is not useful in that individual. A different individual, however, might respond favorably. The overall response in any population, therefore, is dependent on the ratio of responsive to unresponsive individuals. Since personalized medical management is still unavailable, doctors rely on "population medicine" in hopes that the individual patient they are treating is similar to those in the population studied. If that population excluded or failed to include adequate numbers of individuals with genetic features that could influence their responses to the treatment, then how could a population result be applied to an unrepresented individual? If women were excluded or Asians were unrepresented in the study, for instance, how could a drug be approved for everyone?

In the case of BiDil, that reasoning was particularly valid because prior studies had demonstrated that blacks benefited more from the drug than whites. There was also compelling data from other research that black patients are particularly deficient in nitric oxide, the normal cellular constituent that is generated by BiDil. Furthermore, the FDA had given the company an "approvable" letter that stated they would approve the drug if a new study demonstrated benefit in blacks. The A-HeFT study demonstrated in dramatic fashion the benefit in this population. It wasn't one-size-fits-all medicine. For whatever reason we had found a population very responsive to BiDil. The complex mechanisms influencing cardiovascular disease weren't fully understood, but this mechanism in this population was. If the study were also to include a presumably less-responsive non-black population, we had estimated that we would need at least twice as many patients to test the hypothesis. Since our funds were limited it was an easy decision to confine the trial to blacks.

Funding to perform clinical trials is hard to obtain. Their costs are directly related to the number of patients recruited and the complexity of the studies to be performed. The monitoring, data collection and data analysis add to the costs. Trials like A-HeFT may cost as much as $200 million. Government support from the National Institutes of Health is never adequate, and in recent years has become much less available. Pharmaceutical company or device company support is the preferred source, but a study understandably must be able to to provide the sponsor with a marketable treatment if successful. In our case, a small pharmaceutical company seeking its first marketed product had raised the capital to fund A-HeFT.

After approval of the drug some black activists were incensed that the FDA was embracing the view that blacks are "different." Their dedication to eliminating racial categorization in social intercourse blinded them to the possibility that race, however crudely defined, could serve as a valuable biological tool to improve the precision of medical therapy.

Never addressed in the discussion or in the approval process was the question of how to define "blacks". In the study it was solely by self-designation. We all know that is a flawed method to identify a biological marker, if such a marker exists, because racial intermixing is so ubiquitous in America. Who is black was left to the discretion of the doctor and the patient.

Another unusual feature of this approval process was that it was the fourth time the FDA had to make a decision about the approval of this drug combination for heart failure. It was the third time I had presented the data to the Advisory Committee, that group of academic experts appointed to advise the FDA on the safety and effectiveness of drugs developed by the pharmaceutical industry. The first time had been in 1985, four years after my term as chairman of this Advisory Committee and 20 years before the Committee meeting in Gaithersburg and the eventual approval of BiDil. Although records are not kept of such experiences, this may be the longest interval in FDA history between the application for a new drug and its eventual approval.

The story of the discovery, development and testing of BiDil provides a window into clinical cardiovascular research during the past 50 years. The story involves pre-clinical and clinical science, clinical research conduct, regulatory affairs, politics, corporate strategy, racial prejudice, and health care policy. It addresses in depth the world's most prevalent and lethal cardiovascular conditions: hypertension, myocardial infarction, heart failure and shock. It encompasses the effort to develop treatment for advanced symptomatic disease as well as the growing emphasis on preventing early disease from progressing and causing symptoms.

I have been involved in this story since 1956, when I first made observations that ultimately led to BiDil. I have been quoted as saying I felt "vindicated". Reporters have marveled at my "perseverance." But I have been following a path that I knew would eventually be confirmed. It has always been my view that if a disease process is understood it should be possible to treat it effectively. This attitude had its origins in my dealings as a young physician with patients dying from shock, a dramatic and devastating failure of the circulation. I was convinced that insight into the physiologic mechanisms underlying shock could lead to successful therapy that was not being employed properly nor in a timely fashion. BiDil—a compound that beneficially relaxed both arteries and veins and improved the function of the heart—was a product of that physiologic approach to restoring the circulation. So I viewed the approval of BiDil by the FDA more as a vindication of my long-term commitment to understanding and treating mechanisms of disease than of my development of this specific drug.

The approval of BiDil for treatment specifically in blacks with heart failure was not, as trumpeted by Jonathan Kahn in his recent and hysterical book, *Race in a Bottle,* an unethical maneuver by a greedy pharmaceutical company. It was instead the result of a rational pursuit of scientific data that Kahn, in his zeal to discredit the process, has chosen to disregard. Kahn and others have spoken out against the whole idea that racial designation, by whomever it is made, is a useful surrogate for a biological process. Of course we would prefer to have a more sensitive and specific marker for who will benefit, but it does not presently exist. Can the individual's genetic profile serve to identify responders? We are far from that future nirvana when all issues of individual health can supposedly be addressed by the human genome. The fact is that BiDil, given to self-designated blacks with heart failure, prevented 43% of their deaths and kept them out of the hospital. Kahn may complain that white patients were not included, but assigns the wrong reasons to their omission. It is likely that the drug will be effective in a non-black population, but it has yet to be tested. It is irrefutably true, however, that the drug is saving lives in a large and clearly identifiable black population. Even if this population is not biologically homogeneous, it has generally not responded well to other current therapies for heart failure. It is a population in urgent need of effective therapy.

My desire to counter the hostility of Kahn and other critics is one reason for my telling this story. But more important is the harm done by this criticism. The backlash against BiDil has contributed to the woeful infrequency with which the drug is being prescribed. It pains me to know how many black patients with heart failure are dying unnecessarily because they are not taking the drug. Kahn and his acolytes imply that dividing patients by an imperfect effort at racial designation is inherently prejudiced. Their "political correctness" actually is more prejudicial because it is depriving black patients of effective therapy.

The story of the development and testing of BiDil goes far beyond the use of this drug for heart failure. It involves elucidation of the mechanisms and treatment of all cardiovascular diseases that afflict so many of us and will eventually kill more than half of the American population. It also has led to my current interest in preventing cardiovascular disease. If we understand the nature of the processes leading to advanced cardiovascular disease, why can't we apply this knowledge to earlier stages of the disease, when people have not yet become symptomatic? Couldn't early detection of abnormalities in the arteries and heart allow us to intervene to prevent their progression? Heart attacks, strokes and heart failure are usually a consequence of structural changes in the walls of the arteries nourishing the heart and the brain, or of the heart muscle. These abnormalities can be identified long before they result in illnesses that disable or kill us. Why can't we be free from cardiovascular disease, or at least why can't the disease be delayed until people have lived a full life? Everything I have learned in 50years of clinical research has convinced me that this is possible.

My insights over the past half-century have often placed me at odds with colleagues who more closely hew to conventional wisdom. When I dine out with friends, my companions often wonder at my apparent disdain for heart-healthy foods. How, they ask, can a cardiologist eat *foie gras*, steak and buttered rolls? My apparent dietary indiscretion does not reflect disagreement with the role of diet in cardiovascular health, but rather a recognition that it is only one of many factors, both hereditary and environmental, that may be involved. Traditional views often overemphasize diet and interfere with quality of life. My occasional indulgence does not create any personal anxiety. I don't regularly eat a high fat diet, and I usually opt for olive oil instead of butter. Yet the American pre-occupation with the distribution of calories in the diet represents, I believe, an over-emphasis on environment as a cause of atherosclerosis, a build-up of plaque on the walls of arteries. Indeed, a recent study of 4000 year-old mummies found that atherosclerosis was common in 40-year-olds of that era. A modern life-style, it seems, is not a prerequisite for premature atherosclerosis.

Maintaining normal body weight, not smoking, and exercising are very good for you. A sensible and prudent diet is helpful. These lifestyle choices have a significant but modest statistical effect on the frequency of heart attacks and strokes in a population who share one lifestyle choice versus another. The influence on individual risk, however, is highly dependent on other factors that are largely inherited but still not quantifiable. To advocate a so-called "ideal diet" for everyone (including half the population that is not destined to suffer life-altering cardiovascular disease) may serve population medicine but is incompatible with a goal of providing individualized health care.

Drugs are a powerful protector of the arteries and heart, whether the disease is precipitated by genetics or environment. They should be targeted specifically for those at risk. I have now reached an age older and healthier than anyone in my parents' families. I inherited a high risk for heart disease and strokes, but I have been faithfully taking effective medication to protect my arteries and heart for years. My forebears had no access to such drugs.

The process of scientific discovery, as chronicled in this book, is not a linear one. Current concepts may need to be rejected before new ones can take their place. This sometimes requires an attack against conventional wisdom. Such contrarian thinking generates ideas that come at strange times. I have found that the most creative times are those when one is isolated from the daily world and the environment that fosters conformity. The interval between wakefulness and sleep is particularly creative time for me. The shower often provides an interval for creative thinking. Although these moments have often clarified my thinking and been a rich source of new concepts, it is frustrating when these evanescent thoughts cannot be recalled later. I have tried capturing these moments by keeping a pad of paper nearby, but afterward I could never decipher my cryptic notes . I am convinced that many of my best ideas have been lost. Those that remained form the basis of this book.

My long quest to understand and treat cardiovascular disease has been accomplished with a host of colleagues, staff and trainees who have contributed immensely to data collection, interpretation and ideas. Many are identified in the historical account. None of these accomplishments would have been possible without the emotional and physical support of my wife, Syma, and my children, Cynthia, Lauren and Joshua, who put up with an absent and often distracted husband and father during many of those years.

No personal historical account can be entirely factual. Memory is notoriously unreliable. Placing into perspective long-past events, thoughts, and interactions can lead to distortions which could credit me with knowing things that I only learned later. I have tried to avoid this potentially self-serving recitation as I recount the events that surrounded the discoveries reported here. My 750 scientific publications have served to document the sequence of observations and my interpretation of their meaning. The only intentional distortion is of patient's names, which have been altered to protect their privacy.

The challenge in reporting my observations and scientific discoveries has been to make the story accessible to both lay and scientific readers. One might appropriately ask why I have tried to reach both audiences. I am reminded of a painful college rebuke. I decided to take an advanced philosophy seminar class in my senior year, even though I had taken none of the prerequisites for the course. I was confident in my ability, and the highly regarded professor permitted me to join the class. There were seven or eight philosophy majors in the class and the discussions alluded to philosophers whose work I didn't know and to books I had not read. I was clearly in a foreign discipline. Our term paper assignment was to analyze critically a rather complex treatise heavily endowed with what I can best describe as philosophical jargon. The professor, aware of my plans for the medical profession, gave me a B- on my submitted paper and wrote, in what I interpreted as a monumental put-down, "I predict that you will have a successful career interpreting complex medical principles for lay people."

But maybe it wasn't a rebuke. I recently attended an American Heart Association gala at which I received an award for my research. After the dinner and ceremony a woman came up to me and introduced herself. "You lectured to our mini-medical school about 20 years ago", she said. "I loved your talk. You made it so understandable. I have never forgotten how you explained hypertension and heart attacks. It has helped me over the years to deal with illnesses in my family and friends."

The mini-medical school was an effort by the University of Minnesota to engage the lay community by providing a series of lectures designed to educate them about various aspects of medicine. They even received "diplomas" in a mock graduation. As I turned away from her a middle aged man approached. "You won't remember me," he said, "but I was a second-year medical student at the University in 1985. You gave us our cardiology lectures and they are what stimulated me to pursue cardiology as a career."

Perhaps the effort at educating both a professional and lay audience should not be denigrated. The gap between the two appears to be both wider and narrower than one might think. I recently participated in an advisory panel discussion on health literacy among the lay population. A research team had carried out focus group interviews. To their surprise they found that most well-educated and highly intelligent people actually had no idea what blood pressure numbers or cholesterol numbers actually represent, even though they were convinced of their importance. They also were confused about conditions like heart failure. Medical people are familiar with these numbers and diseases, so the gap is wide. But when it comes to a rational way to understand and apply management strategies to these measurements and conditions, doctors often harbor outmoded views that need to be unlearned. Revising pre-conceived misperceptions is often more difficult than learning something new. The gap between the medical and lay audience may be narrower than one might have thought. I have tried to address both audiences with the hope that I have alienated neither.

I have always seemed to function at the interface of two worlds. My philosophy professor put me between the professional and lay audience where I am comfortable. As an academic, he was dedicated to creating a cognoscenti, not informing the masses. As a health care provider, I have always been interested in informing my patients as well as the professionals. My career has also often placed me between the basic scientists and the clinicians. In my early research days I was viewed by clinicians as a basic scientist and by basic scientists as a clinician. *Acceptable to neither* might have been the prediction of my philosophy professor. *Acceptable to both* might have been my long-term goal. *Acceptable to all*—basic scientist, clinician, layman—may be a hill too steep to climb, but the effort is worthwhile.

No one should think that an historical account means the journey has ended. A few years ago I received a "Lifetime Achievement Award" from a prestigious American society. In accepting the award I reminded the assemblage of the Maine farmer who met an inquisitive tourist. "Have you lived here all your life?" she said. "Not yet," he answered quietly.

So the quest goes on. Cardiovascular disease still exists and will eventually result in the death of most of us, both men and women. Our research has helped convince me that progression of the abnormalities that lead to cardiovascular disease can be prevented or at least delayed. Early detection of these abnormalities is now possible and new treatments are being developed to halt their progression to heart attacks, strokes, heart failure, kidney failure, dementia and other cardiovascular diseases. These are all characterized as cardiovascular morbid events. A future without such morbid events interrupting our productive lives is now within our reach. Achieving this goal is a mission I must and will continue to pursue as long as I can.

PROLOGUE

"You learn most from your patients," a professor told our third year medical school class at Cornell in 1954. That was hyperbole, I thought. How could that be true? We were surrounded by faculty, textbooks and medical journals. Certainly these would be our primary sources of knowledge for diagnosing and treating the medical problems we would be facing. The patient would be our focus of attention, I surmised, but not the origin of our knowledge.

It wasn't long after starting my internship at the Beth Israel Hospital in Boston before the truth of the professor's statement became apparent. My first new patient was one whose course not only generated vital questions but who probably determined my entire career. Furthermore, the questions his illness raised in my mind were not addressed by faculty or textbooks. These sources taught what they knew, but generally failed to mention what wasn't known. I discovered that so-called experts are far more interested in what they think they know than in what appears to be unknown. It was this patient whose disease progression fostered my insights into the management of heart attacks (myocardial infarctions), that catastrophic end-stage condition called shock, and that chronic debilitating disease called heart failure. These are diseases or syndromes whose management I have struggled over the years to modernize and refine. This patient also stimulated my understanding of the condition called hypertension, and the mechanisms by which blood pressure and other risk factors precipitate the myocardial infarctions we were trying to treat. He also initiated the thought processes that led to my current dedication to preventing rather than treating advanced heart disease.

What I could not know, of course, was that these questions, and the data generated from our clinical studies, would lead to the development of a new drug, BiDil, and to considerations of individual and ethnic differences in disease responses that would receive Food and Drug Administration approval of the first drug aimed at a single racial group.

I certainly could not have suspected that my research would make me a target of attacks by some sociologists, anthropologists and community activists who claimed that studying ethnic differences was inherently racist.

In July 1956, none of this was in my mind as a stretcher carrying Sam Farber was rolled onto my ward at the Beth Israel Hospital the day after I had begun my internship in Boston. He came from the emergency room where he had been given oxygen and morphine for what he described as crushing chest pain, "like a heavy weight on my chest". The electrocardiogram, recorded in the ER, was handed to me by the orderly who was pushing the stretcher. It showed the characteristic changes of acute and extensive injury to the front or anterior wall of his heart, the worst kind of heart attack. The tracing showed marked elevation of the junction between the electrical signal of the heart's contraction (called the QRS complex) and the subsequent recovery phase (ST segment). This was a sign that the injury had just occurred. It was in its acute phase. Having just graduated from a medical school that was strong on theory but weak on practicality, I felt certain of the diagnosis and its implication for prognosis but less confident than some of my fellow interns in management. Many of them seemed well-versed in what to do in any emergency situation. They even carried in their pockets little guide books which outlined the conventional management strategies for acute illnesses. I had never bought such a book. My anxiety rose as I saw the electrocardiogram tracing. I was now responsible for taking care of this seriously ill patient.

I looked at the man on the stretcher. He was sweating profusely and drowsy from the morphine, his graying wisps of hair matted on his head.

An oxygen mask covered his nose and mouth and the oxygen tank was being pushed by a nurse's aide. In the ER, he had been put in a hospital gown tied loosely at the neck so that tufts of black and gray chest hair peeped out above the sheet covering him. His wife held his hand as she walked alongside the stretcher, bending periodically to kiss his moist forehead. Her dark hair was pulled back in a bun and she was carefully dressed, looking like a woman accustomed to being in control of her environment. Sam and Naomi Farber would forever be a part of my life.

Beth Israel Hospital in Boston was one of the country's most coveted medicine internships. It was a primary teaching hospital of Harvard Medical School, and its faculty was considered to be among the best. My fellow interns were all honors graduates of leading medical schools, many from Harvard. Beth Israel, like many "Jewish" hospitals in the country, was initially organized to provide a hospital for Jewish doctors who could not gain access to the staffs of other private hospitals. Over time, however, these hospitals, as well as the previously discriminatory ones, became essentially non-sectarian and provided access to all doctors and all patients. Many Jewish patients, like Sam Farber, chose Beth Israel as their hospital of choice, but neither the interns nor staff paid much attention to religion or race.

The ward service at Beth Israel consisted of a large open room with about 15 beds arranged against the walls. Our job as interns was to admit patients to that service, under the supervision of a resident and staff physician, and to make ward rounds at least twice daily by walking from bed to bed along with a nurse and an unwieldy rolling chart rack. We were assigned for 6 weeks at a time to the ward service. The problem we were warned of by the previous interns, who now were beginning their residency, was that patient turnover was low. Since our goal as interns was to learn as much as possible by seeing a variety of diseases, low turnover meant a deficient education.

One of the main reasons for the low turnover was myocardial infarction. The consensus was that these patients were not very interesting but would occupy a bed for more than a month while they recovered.

They would prevent us from admitting more interesting and instructive patients to our service. The problem was so serious that we made it the focus of the annual skit that the interns perform every Spring to entertain their more senior colleagues. We composed a parody on the Gilbert and Sullivan *HMS Pinafore* song "I'm Called Little Buttercup." Our song ended "...and if I find parked here, another infarct here, I'll either go daft or go home." This little parody, along with a number of other modified songs, was a feature of the light-hearted effort designed to make fun of ourselves and the hospital staff. Such efforts at satire reached their zenith some years later when another intern, Stephen Bergman, using a pseudonym wrote a far more scathing parody on Beth Israel health care in a coveted best seller called "The House of God."

Myocardial infarction, or heart attack, was viewed as a waste of time for an intern. The damage to the heart muscle or myocardium had already occurred before we saw the patient and there was nothing to do but "baby-sit", to protect the patient from some undescribed bad event while the damaged or infarcted area in the muscle was forming a stable scar. That meant up to six weeks occupying a precious bed on our ward before it was "safe" to let the patient depart in a wheelchair to complete their slow convalescence at home. Of course, it was not known that myocardial infarction (MI) is caused by a blood clot in the coronary artery, not by cholesterol-containing plaques gradually obstructing the artery. Or that the coronary artery can be opened by emergent angioplasty with a balloon. Or that the clot can be dissolved by prompt injection of a clot-dissolving drug when the patient is first seen. The only urgent therapy we employed was morphine to relieve pain.

In retrospect, I am not certain what we thought had caused the acute episode of damage to the heart muscle or myocardium. Doctors were apparently more interested in dealing with the patient than exploring the mechanism. According to conventional wisdom, the coronary artery nourishing the muscle had become occluded so the blood flow to that area of the muscle ceased. In subsequent years, however, pathologists noted the absence at autopsy of clots in the coronary arteries. This was taken as evidence against sudden occlusion of blood flow by a thrombus or clot. (We now know that many clots dissolve by themselves after the damage is done.)

Atherosclerotic cholesterol plaques were always present in the patients' coronary arteries, but why did they obstruct so suddenly? Some proposed that the coronary artery might go into spasm to obstruct blood flow. Others sought subtle metabolic explanations not related to obstruction for the injury. A wide range of theories existed about what caused MI's in patients with plaques in their coronary arteries. Coronary atherosclerosis, or plaques, was viewed as a chronic disease, but it was a mystery why it precipitated an acute event (MI) at the time it did. None of the theories had been substantiated and the mystery seemed so hard to solve that textbooks and teachers largely disregarded the issue.

Each intern had about eight patients on whom we made detailed rounds at least twice daily with intermediate visits frequently during the day and night—we spent every other night on-call in the hospital. Over a six-week convalescence we would get to know the patients and their families more intimately than their best friends. Personal concerns such as food fetishes, bowel habits, financial stresses, family crises and individual anxieties became part of the daily interaction. When families were close, the interaction between intern and spouse became almost as intense as that between intern and patient. The tradition was not to share details of the illness with the patient for fear he or she would become dangerously stressed. Instead, we shared this information with the spouse and other family members. That practice has dramatically changed in the current era of full disclosure to patients and limited disclosure to others.

After Sam Farber had been carefully moved from the stretcher to the only vacant bed on the ward, I pulled up a chair, and began taking a history. He was the first new patient of my internship, but I wanted to appear experienced, not letting my apprehension show. He was still groggy from the morphine and still having pressure in his chest, he said, but was remarkably anxious to be cooperative. Naomi sat at the end of the bed appearing more anxious than he was. Sam was a pharmacist. He was 61, had smoked for a number of years (Naomi didn't like the smell and had urged him for years to stop) and he had been noted by his physician to have high blood pressure or hypertension for the past 10 years. Treatment for high blood pressure was controversial in those days. Some advocated drug treatment, but the drugs were not very effective and had a number of side effects. Other experts felt it was dangerous to lower blood pressure, perhaps because the high pressure might be necessary to deliver adequate blood to the tissues. These experts avoided treatment to lower blood pressure unless the pressure had risen to very high levels that were clearly damaging the kidneys, brain or heart, a condition called malignant hypertension. It was some years before their approach was discredited by well-designed clinical trials. As a pharmacist Sam was aware of this controversy, and he occasionally took a drug called reserpine when he thought his pressure was too high. He had a blood pressure cuff in his drug store and learned how to take his own blood pressure, especially when he felt stressed.

He had had no symptoms of heart trouble prior to this acute event, which had started about 5 A.M. that morning when he awoke with a vague sensation of pressure in his chest. Naomi had told him to stay in bed while she dressed and then went to the kitchen to prepare breakfast. By the time she returned to the bedroom he was sweating profusely and in obvious pain. An ambulance was called and brought him to the Beth Israel ER. Nothing else in his history seemed particularly pertinent at the time.

What struck me from the first moment I met Sam and Naomi was their closeness and respect for each other. Naomi was a school teacher. School was closed for the summer and she spent every day—all day—with Sam in the hospital. She never really smiled. I couldn't tell if this was due to a life-long pattern of austerity or a consequence of his illness. After Sam had stabilized and was beginning his recovery he was moved from the open ward to a semi-private room. Although visiting hours were limited we made an exception for Naomi because their closeness and their uncommon sensitivity made them ward favorites. Their two children—both grown and with families of their own—displayed the same warmth during their long visits. They were all usually at Sam's bedside during my evening rounds.

I couldn't help comparing Sam's family with my own, which hadn't spent much time while I was growing up sitting around having substantive discussions like the Farber family apparently did. We rarely experienced animated interaction during family gatherings, but such conversation was common when I visited Sam's bedside with his family present. My father was working in his upstairs den most evenings. He was an important man in Schenectady, N.Y., having served as the City Engineer and then as City Manager. He also edited an engineering journal that seemed to consume most of his evenings and weekends. My mother was a patient listener, quick to render an opinion. She became the advisor to aunts, uncles and acquaintances who came to the house to seek her counsel. My sister, more than five years older than me, often carried on conversations with my mother that didn't interest me. I didn't seek advice. Rather than conversing with me, my mother tried to help and my father was judgmental. There was not much overt expression of warmth. The Farber family, on the other hand, seemed to love each other unconditionally. I wondered what it would have been like to grow up in their family.

Of course I now had the beginnings of a family of my own. Syma Cheris, who grew up in Albany about 15 miles away, had become my girlfriend while I was in college. She went to New York University as an English major after high school graduation and I followed her to New York to attend Cornell University Medical School the next year. We got married after my first year of medical school and moved into a small, unheated (except for a kerosene space heater) railroad apartment on East 70th Street near Cornell. We shared it with some large cockroaches and an occasional rodent. But the price was right—$26 a month. After graduation she got a publishing job to help support us. Now that I was an intern, I was getting paid $25 a month, and Syma had found a job in

Boston not quite to her liking, but at least it provided a pay check. We had rented an apartment in Back Bay, a few blocks from the hospital. We certainly were not yet ready for children, but I knew the time would come. The Farber family seemed to be a good model for our future family.

Over the ensuing six weeks, Sam made what appeared to be an uncomplicated recovery. Prior to his heart attack he had been completely dedicated to his drug store and to his customers, who depended on him for all sorts of medical and non-medical advice. On my frequent late evening visits to his bedside he expressed concern about my long hours and often gave more attention to me than I paid to him. In the third week, when he began to think he would survive, he started talking about selling the drugstore, a decision that Naomi was reluctant to support because she feared he would become depressed without it.

I viewed his recovery and watched his resolving electrocardiographic changes (nearly daily electrocardiograms were about the only test we had in those days) and decided he should do well. There was no coronary angiography in 1956 to document the severity of coronary disease, and no coronary surgery or angioplasty or stents to bypass blockages. There was no echocardiography, the ultrasound technique we now utilize to assess the size and function of the heart's left ventricle that is damaged by the infarction. There were no drugs to alter the course of the disease, which was left to its own natural history.

Sam appeared to be doing well. I urged him to keep his store and return to work in a few months, at a time when the scar in his heart muscle should be firm enough for him to safely resume productive activity. It had always been my bias that people should not give in to disease. While a medical student, I had seen patients become self-proclaimed cripples for illnesses that I thought should not have been disabling. I didn't want Sam and Naomi to become victims of this psychological disability. This was one of my first encounters with an in-depth doctor-patient relationship. I found the experience exhilarating and fulfilling.

When Sam was ready to be discharged I ordered a chest x-ray and electrocardiogram. His heart size appeared normal. Even his blood pressure was now normal. It was well known that after a heart attack previously hypertensive patients often experience normalization of their blood pressure, at least temporarily. He had been out of bed for over a week with brief walks around the ward and two trips down to the hospital lobby with Naomi. He had no symptoms to suggest inadequacy of coronary blood flow and no shortness of breath to suggest that his heart was not pumping effectively. My advice was to walk around the house for two weeks, with one trip per day up to the second floor, and then to begin walking outside. We planned a careful rehabilitation program so that on the fifth week at home he could begin going into the store for an hour a day, gradual increasing this activity until he could begin working a full day by the fourth month after his heart attack.

Diet and smoking were not important issues in those days. Many of the interns smoked in our house staff lounge. I consulted my medical school "bible", *Harrison's Textbook of Medicine*, to read the expert's view of appropriate medical advice for patients when leaving the hospital after a myocardial infarction. Tinsley Harrison, the editor of the book and a revered figure in cardiology, had written the chapter. He pointed out that there was no evidence that diet made any difference in long-term management, but did indicate that "some believe that a low-cholesterol diet should be followed permanently…" Regarding smoking, Harrison's view was remarkable in light of current evidence and practice. He stated: "Smoking in moderation (8 to 12 cigarettes daily) may be allowed in most instances…" Given my desire to support Naomi, and the fact that Sam had not smoked in the hospital, I urged him to abandon the habit.

We shook hands as he left and his hand lingered in mine before he withdrew it. I noticed his eyes were moist. Perhaps mine were, too. I kissed Naomi. I didn't know if it was appropriate for a doctor to kiss a patient's wife, but I had developed a fondness for her steadfastness and caring. She was still unsmiling but appeared to be back in control, her hair carefully pulled back and her posture straight. She was obviously anxious to put this episode behind her and return to the life she knew. I would miss them. During the first month of my internship they had become my Beth Israel family.

My medical care for Sam was complete, I thought. His bed could now be occupied by a more interesting medical problem, and I would soon be moving on to a new service for my second six-week assignment.

Six months later, when I was back on the ward for another rotation, I encountered Sam and Naomi again. Once again, Sam was on a stretcher coming from the ER with Naomi at his side. He was not having chest pain this time but was profoundly short of breath. He was propped up on the stretcher with three big pillows and wore an oxygen mask that kept falling off. Naomi was mopping his drenched forehead. He was in what we called fulminant heart failure with pulmonary edema, a condition in which the lungs fill with fluid because the pumping ability of the heart is severely impaired.

Naomi's recitation of the events leading up to this acute problem was of little help. He had done exactly as told and had been followed closely by his private doctor. He had gone back to work two months before and complained only of fatigue and some shortness of breath when climbing stairs, symptoms that we might well have attributed to deconditioning from the prolonged inactivity. He had developed some ankle puffiness in the past two weeks, a sign of fluid retention that would have alerted us to the possibility that his heart's weakening pumping might be reducing the ability of the kidneys to excrete salt. The day before his ER visit, he had become more short of breath and began coughing up white sputum. The doctor had administered a mercurial diuretic, the drug we used at that time to help the kidney rid the body of excess fluid, but the symptoms worsened.

I will never forget the faces of Sam and Naomi that morning as they arrived on the ward. Sam had a look of resignation, an apparent sense that all was now lost. He wanted me to say that he would be okay, that his condition could easily be treated, but he knew that wasn't true. Naomi, on the other hand, stood in judgment. Her eyes implored me to explain why this had happened despite following my detailed instructions, She had subtly placed me on trial. At that moment she looked more like my father than like Naomi Farber.

An electrocardiogram showed no new changes, but a chest x-ray revealed a markedly enlarged heart with pulmonary edema, the fluffy infiltrates that appear when fluid is blocking the lung's ability to exchange oxygen for carbon dioxide. On examination his lungs exhibited the bubbling sounds we associate with fluid all the way up to the top of the lungs. The jugular veins in his neck were bulging to above the angle of the jaw, a sure sign of heart failure.

My resident and I applied tourniquets to all four extremities to obstruct the draining veins and trap blood in the arms and legs to unburden the heart. We gave diuretics and digitalis—all the medical treatment known at that time. During the next 48 hours I didn't leave the hospital, and neither did Naomi. I had trouble looking at her. I was failing.

What had happened to Sam?

I asked my resident and my attending physician professor. I asked the staff cardiologists. I asked a famous cardiologist, Sam Levine, from a neighboring institution. Why should this man, who had left the hospital five months ago with a normal-sized and apparently normally functioning heart, now have severe heart failure? He probably had more heart damage, perhaps another infarct, I was told. But he had had no new chest pain and his electrocardiogram was unchanged. New heart damage should have shown up on the electrocardiogram. Perhaps he had suffered pulmonary emboli, those clots that break off in the legs and go to the lung, I was told. But he was in left heart failure and that would cause right heart failure, I pleaded. Perhaps he had a subtle infection, I was told. But there was no fever, no elevation of white blood cell count, and no signs of organ involvement that would be signs of infection.

Nobody could tell me why Sam Farber had developed heart failure.

I have always been interested in the mechanism of events. My view was that all things that happen can be explained if only we could understand them. In medical school I could never memorize lists. I insisted instead on understanding how each thing on the list operated. I wanted to know how it got there, what the evidence was, how it was discovered, how sound were the data. My first year cadaver partner, the person I spent hours with each day dissecting opposite sides of a body, was a devout Mormon. Contrary to my view, he believed that God's plan for him would determine his life and that science could not influence that plan or anyone's life. He flunked out after the first year.

Here in my internship I came to realize that lack of interest in mechanisms was more widespread than just in my lab partner. Lack of interest in discovery was even more pervasive. A certain medical publication seemed to establish "fact" without much inquiry into the observations and methods used in the investigation. There seemed to be little awareness that today's "facts", if casually accepted, could turn out to be fiction tomorrow.

Most of my colleagues loved to read the scientific literature to match up published observations with their own. If there were no publications the problem did not exist. Few if any authors had addressed the issue of why the heart failed months after a myocardial infarction (MI). Most of the doctors at Harvard were comfortable with the status quo. Heart failure after MI had to be fit into what was already known. The heart muscle was damaged by the MI—the heart failed. This was not particularly interesting to them.

The next two days with Sam and Naomi were hectic. His condition deteriorated progressively despite our therapeutic efforts. Digitalis did not control his accelerating heart rate. He had intermittent bouts of ventricular tachycardia (a potentially fatal heart rhythm disturbance) for which we used the best drug treatments available at that time. (Some of these drugs have now been shown to be paradoxically lethal in this situation.) His blood pressure began to fall, reaching levels where it could not be recorded by the arm cuff, and we diagnosed "shock", a state of inadequate blood flow that is almost always fatal. We used the usual drugs that raise blood pressure by constricting the arteries and stimulating the heart to beat more forcefully, but our feeble attempts were met by worsening pump failure. Sam died with Naomi and his children at his side.

I cried with Naomi, probably as much out of frustration with my ignorance as out of sadness at losing a man, husband and father who had been my first patient and had come to mean so much to me. I had failed and I did not know why. Perhaps myocardial infarction was not as simple a disease as I had been told. We didn't know how to treat any of the conditions that Sam suffered from: hypertension, myocardial infarction, shock, or heart failure. They must all in some way be related, I concluded—but how? I could no longer be complacent. I had to explore the unknown.

It was to be my lifelong mission.

CHAPTER I
Hypertension

One in three U.S. adults has hypertension, according to 2010 data from the American Heart Association. Two-thirds of those over the age of 60 have hypertension. This is a mind-numbing statistic! "What's going on?" you may ask. If it's this common how can it be called a disease? If it is a disease, how is it defined? Why is it so common? What causes it? Does it need to be treated?

I was asking those same questions when I was a medical student in the mid-l950s. I had found hypertension, usually called essential hypertension, fascinating. It's true that my mother had it, a couple of my uncles had it, and the wife of one of my classmates died from a very severe form of it called malignant hypertension while we were in medical school. But it was more than these personal connections that piqued my interest. Maybe it had something to do with my attraction to complex systems.

Blood pressure is a number generated by a complex interaction. The heart pumps into the arteries that lead from the heart and nourish all the organs of the body. When the heart pumps, it generates a pressure much like any pump ejecting into a closed system. This pressure is transmitted into the arteries leading from the heart. The magnitude of the pressure will depend on the rate at which the pump ejects the blood, the amount of blood pumped with each beat, and the resistance to flow imposed by the arterial system into which the heart empties. Is the pressure determined by the pump—that is, the heart—or is the pressure determined by the arterial system? No one to this day fully understands which comes first in the natural history of essential hypertension.

Measuring blood pressure

Early in our medical student training we learned to take blood pressure on each other. We were taught to pump air into a cuff which we had wrapped around the upper arm until the pressure in the cuff, defined on a mercury manometer, was well above the individual's expected blood pressure. At that point blood flow to the arm was blocked by the cuff compressing the artery (the brachial artery), which is the sole source of blood flow to the arm. We then released a valve that allowed the air to leak slowly out of the cuff, listening carefully with a stethoscope placed over the artery just below the cuff as the pressure gradually fell. The first sound, we were told, will signal *systolic pressure*, which represents the pressure during the peak of ejection from the heart. This first sound results from the transient flow of blood during the short interval when the pressure in the brachial artery surpasses the pressure compressing the artery.

As the pressure in the cuff continues to fall, the sounds eventually disappear. This represents the *diastolic pressure*, which is the pressure in the arteries just before the next heartbeat. No sound is generated when the cuff is no longer interfering with blood flow during any portion of the heartbeat.

When we measured blood pressure repeatedly in our fellow students, it was never the same twice. Did it change because the pressure was varying? Did it vary because the output from the heart changed from moment to moment, or because the resistance imposed by the arteries changed? Or did it change because our technique and our hearing were variable? There was no way to find out, but we all suspected that all of the above were involved. So measurement of blood pressure was an inexact methodology, and it hasn't changed since the 1950s when we practiced on our classmates. It's still inexact and variable. It's one of the few things in medicine that has not changed.

Despite all the problems with measuring blood pressure, and despite its marked variability from time to time, this blood pressure measurement was the only way to diagnose the disease called hypertension. I was flabbergasted by the crudeness of the diagnostic technique combined with the rigor of the diagnostic criteria.

Blood pressure measurements are reported in millimeters of mercury (mmHg) because, as noted above, a column of mercury was used in the traditional technique to monitor the amount of pressure in the cuff required to obstruct the artery in the arm. We were told that a diastolic blood pressure greater than 90 mmHg meant that the patient had hypertension.

But if the pressure varied every time I took it, and if I was often uncertain whether the sounds heard over the artery disappeared at 92, 90 or 88 mmHg, how was I to be confident in my diagnosis? We were told to make sure patients were sitting comfortably at rest when we measured the blood pressure. But what if they were nervous, as patients often are? And what if they had just eaten a big meal or climbed three flights of stairs? How were we to factor all those things into our diagnostic effort?

I was puzzled and no one seemed able to help me. They seemed wedded to the numbers, however crude the method of recording them.

It is now more than 50 years later. Certainly we are now better able to deal with these issues and make a more confident diagnosis, aren't we? The answer, unfortunately, is no. We still use the same cuff. We are still plagued by imprecision and variability. Mercury has disappeared from most medical facilities, but the unit of pressure in mmHg has been preserved. Newer instruments now provide a digital read-out of pressures without requiring listening to the sounds over the artery, but the imprecision and variability are no better. Patients often are now asked to buy their own blood pressure cuffs to record their pressures at different times of the day at home. Drug stores and health clubs usually have blood pressure machines for patients to self-record. So almost everyone now knows his or her blood pressure, at least as accurately as the instrument can record it.

What do these pressures mean?

How is hypertension defined?

The diagnostic criteria for hypertension have changed dramatically. The old emphasis on a specific level of diastolic pressure for the diagnosis has largely been replaced by a focus on systolic blood pressure, often with the diastolic pressure simply thrown in. So the criterion for the diagnosis of hypertension is now generally accepted as greater than 140 mmHg systolic or 90 mmHg diastolic. But it's gotten far more complicated. Some experts think that pressures over 130/85 mmHg can also be considered "hypertensive", especially if the patient has diabetes or an elevated blood sugar level. Furthermore, an American consensus panel has concluded that any pressure above 120/80 mmHg places the individual at "higher risk" and therefore has come up with a most confusing term called "prehypertension" to refer to this large population.

Which pressure measurement should we be using to make these diagnoses? The best answer usually provided is that one should average a number of readings to arrive at the precise number on which to make the diagnosis. Fifty years ago that seemed to be a remarkably crude way to make such an important diagnosis.

It still does.

$$\text{Blood Pressure (BP)} = \text{Cardiac Output (CO)} \times \text{Systemic Vascular Resistance (SVR)}$$

Figure I – 1

Blood pressure is a product of cardiac output, the amount of blood pumped by the heart over a given time, and the vascular resistance imposed by the state of constriction on the structure of small arteries throughout the body. In most individuals with hypertension, it is increased vascular resistance that causes the rise in pressure.

It was the general consensus that, since the amount of blood pumped by the heart (cardiac output) is not usually increased in people with established hypertension, elevated blood pressure must be a consequence of a rise in vascular resistance. A rise in resistance means that the small arteries that control blood flow to all the organs of the body are narrowed. Why the small arteries were narrowed was a mystery to me, and apparently a mystery to all the experts whose papers I tried to read. There were too many possible mechanisms to identify any one at fault. In fact, one widely held theory was that the heart itself was the primary cause. The hypothesis, based on serial observations in young individuals with hypertension, was that the heart in certain individuals pumped too hard and ejected more blood than the body needed. In response to this excess blood flow, the small arteries "autoregulated" by narrowing to reduce the unwanted flow. No one really understood how this "autoregulation" occurred, but the standard view was that the artery simply knew when to constrict. Such constriction in many small arteries would raise resistance to blood flow and raise the pressure. The raised pressure, this theory suggested, would tell the heart to reduce its contractions and return its ejected blood flow to normal, but the artery narrowing would persist. The patient now had a condition with a normal cardiac output and a high resistance, the very state observed in most patients with hypertension. That theory has never really been confirmed or refuted. Indeed, no experts are much interested in even debating it, since there are no useful data to analyze.

Genes and hypertension

Since life insurance actuarial data revealed that there was a direct relationship between blood pressure and shortened life expectancy, it was clear that whatever was narrowing the arteries was having adverse consequences. Sam Farber's hypertension, which was poorly treated in those days, may well have had something to do with causing his heart attack. If hypertension shortens your life, then something diabolical is causing the small arteries to be narrowed. And since hypertension tends to occur in families, there is probably some genetic cause that has persisted over the centuries despite its adverse effect on survival.

The process of breeding out adverse genomic trends is called "natural selection" or "survival of the fittest." Mutations or spontaneous changes may occur in an offspring's genetic material. If that change adversely affects early survival, such as increasing the susceptibility to severe infections, then such individuals will be less likely to survive and will not reproduce. The mutation over generations will gradually disappear from the population. On the other hand, if the mutation has a beneficial effect on survival, such as resistance to infection, the mutation will be passed on and gradually increase its prevalence in the population.

The complexity of this process is best exemplified by sickle cell disease, which is a common cause of anemia and death in Africa. How did the genetic trait for sickle cell disease become common in Africa and so rare elsewhere? Sickle cell disease is caused by a mutation in the hemoglobin gene that leads to misshapen red blood cells. If one has the bad luck to have inherited a mutated gene from both parents, the result is the full-blown disease with severe complications and a shortened life. In most parts of the world this adverse survival effect has resulted in a gradual disappearance of the mutation.

In Africa, however, malaria swept through the population for thousands of years and killed millions of children and adults. The gene for sickle cell disease did not disappear in this part of the world because the abnormal red blood cell protected the affected individual from the ravages of malaria, which is caused by a parasite that grows in normal red blood cells but not in those harboring the mutated gene. Indeed, the abnormal gene is protective from malaria even in individuals who have inherited only one such mutation—from either mother or father, but not both. Those individuals have no symptoms of their sickle cell trait but are protected from malaria. So having a mutant gene in Africa is protective, and the abnormality therefore persisted and proliferated.

What about hypertension? If it is such a powerful cause of heart attacks and strokes, why hasn't the gene for hypertension—if there is one—disappeared over thousands of years? Most experts believe there must be gene patterns or other identifiable hereditary markers that define individuals who will develop hypertension. It is certainly not a single gene, as in sickle cell disease. Hypertension's persistence, and perhaps even its increasing prevalence, over the centuries may suggest that it could have some as yet unidentified protective effect.

On the other hand, the complications and mortality from hypertension mainly affects individuals who are beyond their procreative years. The presence of hypertension does not reduce the fertility of the people affected, so the natural selection process cannot operate. Therefore, hypertension, which clearly is related to both hereditary and environmental factors, continues to proliferate in our society.

What causes hypertension?

I was so interested in hypertension during medical school that I made it the subject of my senior thesis, a research paper that was required for graduation at Cornell. I pored through the literature and became fascinated with the physiologic abnormalities of the circulation that had been detected in hypertension. Abnormalities in the arteries and the heart, disturbances of the kidneys and brain, alterations in the nervous system—these were all elegantly described in experimental animals and humans. No one, however, really dealt with the arbitrariness of the diagnosis of this disease. Since blood pressure measurement was the only means of diagnosis, the question was at what level of pressure is the diagnosis made.

During my medical school days, that level was usually defined as 160 over 100 mmHg or above. In more recent years that number has gradually fallen to the point that the most recent government committee on management of hypertension defined levels below 120 over 80 as normal; anything above can be classified as either prehypertension or hypertension. Clearly we were confused in the 1950s—and maybe even more confused today. But since the majority of middle-aged and elderly people have systolic pressures over 120 mmHg, we have defined a majority of the aging population as abnormal. Should we be proud of that or astounded by it?

A debate about hypertension developed in the early 1960s between George Pickering and Robert Platt, two British investigators who were knighted by the Queen. Pickering claimed that blood pressure was normally distributed throughout the population. That is, like all variables such as height, there was a range of values in any population from low to high, with fewer individuals at the low and high ends and the majority in the middle. The frequency distribution takes the form of the well-known bell-shaped curve (Figure I-2).

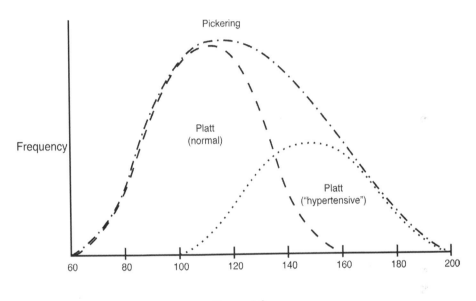

Figure I-2

The proposed distribution of systolic blood pressures in a population. Pickering viewed it as a single population. Platt proposed that there were two separate populations, each with its own distribution of pressures. Since blood pressures overlapped, separating hypertensives from normals would therefore require some measurement other than blood pressure.

According to Pickering's view, hypertension existed in that population that was at the upper end of the blood pressure distribution curve. It was not critical where you placed the threshold for hypertension on the distribution curve because, wherever you separated the normals from the hypertensives, you would identify a subset of the population with higher pressures and higher risk for cardiovascular disease. If heredity was involved, Pickering concluded that its expression was in the blood pressure itself. Therefore, *the blood pressure is the disease.* It is merely the higher end of a normal blood pressure distribution in the population.

Platt's view was quite different. He thought that the distribution curve in populations was not symmetrical, but that there was a bulge at the higher end that suggested a different population with slightly higher pressures. Hypertension, in his view, was not the higher end of a normal distribution, but a different population that had inherited "hypertension". This population had its own distribution of blood pressures. Those pressures averaged higher than in the normal population (accounting for the bulge on the curves) but largely overlapped the pressures in the normal group (Figure I-2). Platt didn't think that elevated blood pressure was the disease, but rather a manifestation of the disease. Unfortunately, he had no way to identify the disease. The medical community, largely uninterested in the debate, continued to use the blood pressure cuff to diagnose the disease.

My first contact with George Pickering was anything but satisfying. He was a revered professor of medicine at Oxford. His appearance in 1959 to give a lecture at the University of Texas in Galveston, where I was fulfilling my military obligation at a Public Health Service Hospital, was certainly a special event. He had already been knighted, so the aura of Sir George's appearance was further enhanced. I remember his lecture vividly. He described his early experience with the treatment of hypertension. He followed patients with elevated blood pressure until they developed what was called "malignant hypertension", a condition with extremely elevated pressures and severe symptoms associated with organ damage and a short life expectancy. He then proudly displayed the anecdotal results of patients whose blood pressure was lowered in response to his drug therapy. These patients appeared to be clinically improved and they lived somewhat longer, although most succumbed to their disease within months.

It struck me that the optimal time to initiate therapy would have been before they entered the so-called malignant phase of their disease. During the Q&A period after his talk, as senior physicians were congratulating him on his provocative work, I asked why he hadn't considering beginning therapy earlier. He accused me of naiveté for suggesting that drugs to lower blood pressure should be administered to apparently healthy people without symptoms. I received scornful looks from the senior faculty.

Treatment of hypertension

Much has happened in the field since my encounter with Sir George, and much has stayed the same. We now routinely treat elevated blood pressure in adults without symptoms. Although the debate between Pickering and Platt was never fully settled, doctors have remained dependent on diagnosing hypertension by measuring blood pressure. Few investigators have made any attempt to identify another diagnostic tool. This means that blood pressure remains the only appropriate means of separating normal from hypertensive individuals. Since blood pressure values exist as a continuum, as displayed in Figure I- 2, an arbitrary level had to be established to identify those with a "disease". In England, this level was initially set at greater than 160/100 mmHg. In the U.S., lower values of "normal" gradually became accepted and 140/90 mmHg eventually became the worldwide criterion for the diagnosis of hypertension. The "elephant in the room"—the variability issue—was usually disregarded.

The mechanism by which the small arteries narrow in hypertension has never been fully explained. It is now clear, however, that this narrowing represents not only a constriction of the smooth muscle in the arteries, but also a structural change in the small arteries that become thicker and stiffer with a smaller lumen. Treatment is now initiated at a much earlier stage of the disease, and newer blood pressure guidelines now identify a normal blood pressure as less than 120/80 mmHg, a far cry from the days of Sir George. These guidelines advocate aggressive attempts to lower blood pressure in patients with pressures greater than140/90mmHg and are suggesting treating even lower levels in certain high risk individuals.

But the currently advocated approach remains consistent with the Pickering hypothesis—that blood pressure is a product of genes and environment, and that individuals with the higher pressures, wherever the threshold is placed, are the ones who need treatment.

I disagree. I think Platt was right all along. Blood pressure may provide a clue to the disease, but the disease itself is in the small arteries. Many people have early disease in the arteries with blood pressures less than 140/90mmHg. They should probably be treated. Others have blood pressures that may occasionally be elevated, especially in the doctor's office, but have no abnormality of their small arteries; these people probably should not be treated. There are therefore two populations, those with the disease and those without. Blood pressure certainly tends to be higher in those with disease, but blood pressure is an imprecise way to distinguish the groups. We need a diagnostic tool to supplement blood pressure measurement in order to identify hypertension. An innovative approach to this quest will be discussed later.

Challenging conventional wisdom

I was elected by my colleagues in 1996 to serve as President of the International Society of Hypertension (ISH), a large multinational group composed of all the national and regional hypertension societies around the world. They elected me despite my well-known view that blood pressure, the phenomenon they earned their living measuring, was not the disease. The biannual meetings of ISH represent the largest gatherings of hypertension experts in the world. It is traditional for the President to address this gathering. During my presidency the meeting was held in Glasgow.

I remember the Glasgow meeting particularly well. It was the first and last time I wore a kilt, which was provided for me by the Scotch organizers to wear at the gala dinner in honor of my presidency. Fortunately, I was not asked to wear it at the opening scientific session the next morning, where I presented the Presidential Address.

I prepared carefully for my lecture by marshalling evidence to support my thesis that a blood vessel abnormality, not blood pressure, was the key to the disease process. As I stepped off the podium after my lecture I was greeted by an Irish woman physician who hugged me and began crying.

"I have waited years for someone to say what you just said," she cried. "I was afraid I would never hear the truth."

But the response of others was either muted or downright hostile. Some friends shunned me, unwilling to congratulate me but not wanting to confront me. I recognized that the traditional organization I was now leading could not be convinced to revise their concept of hypertension as a blood pressure disease. Nonetheless, the editor of the Society's journal, *Journal of Hypertension*, urged me to submit my lecture for publication. It was published some months later under the title "Arteries, myocardium, blood pressure and cardiovascular risk: towards a revised definition of hypertension". I was pleased with the paper, but it did not inspire a movement to change the diagnostic criteria for hypertension. Only in recent years has a group of colleagues from the American Society of Hypertension, the organization of clinical experts in the United States of which I had also served as President, convened to publish a revised definition of hypertension similar to the one I had proposed in Glasgow.

Stiffening of the arteries

Over the years I became convinced that the hypertensive and normal populations could be distinguished by something other than blood pressure. Rather than relying on the systolic and diastolic pressures obtained by a cuff measurement, we began examining the entire pressure waveform, which could be recorded directly from a needle in an artery or, far more conveniently, with a pressure transducer (a small sensor) placed over an accessible artery, such as the radial artery at the wrist (Figure I- 3).

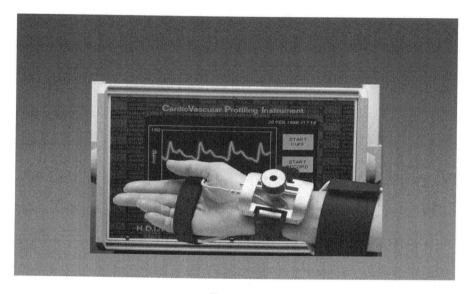

Figure I-3

The sensor is placed over the radial artery at the wrist and held in place by a housing and an arm brace. The recorded waveform is displayed on a video screen. The waveform recorded from the skin is identical to a pressure waveform that could be recorded directly from inside the artery.

These waveforms provide far more information than the systolic pressure peak and the diastolic trough, which were the numbers recorded with a blood pressure cuff on the arm. At the University of Minnesota in the 1990s, my bioengineering colleague Stan Finkelstein and I developed a computer program to analyze these waveforms. With this program and a model system based on an electrical analogue, we were able to separately identify the stiffness of the large and small arteries. Over the past decade we and other investigators have generated data suggesting that stiff small arteries identify the disease of hypertension far more precisely than blood pressure. I even helped found a company, Hypertension Diagnostics, which licensed the technology from the University of Minnesota and now markets this device, the CV Profilor. It is in wide use around the world to assist in the diagnosis and management of hypertension.

A research fellowship

In 1960, however, as I was completing my assignment in Galveston, having finished an internship and a year of medical residency in Boston, I was searching for a research fellowship during which I could pursue my interest in understanding and treating hypertension. The dilemma of Sam Farber's untreated and rapidly progressive disease was still in my mind. I selected a program at Georgetown University in Washington, D.C., supervised by Dr. Edward Freis, one of the first experts in hypertension who appeared to be interested in patient management and was advocating drug treatment of high blood pressure.

Dr. Freis was carrying out the very first clinical trial to determine whether drugs that reduced blood pressure could reduce morbidity and mortality in hypertensive patients. Such a study had not previously been performed and there was still a vocal group of so-called experts who insisted that elevated blood pressure was in some patients a necessary abnormality to provide enough blood flow to organs. These experts suggested that lowering blood pressure could accelerate the occurrence of morbid events. Ed Freis's study finally laid to rest that misinterpretation when the study demonstrated that by administering drugs to lower blood pressure, patients lived longer and had fewer heart attacks and strokes.

My fellowship was dedicated to learning how to do research and learning how to play golf. The research experience was valuable but the golf instruction was questionable. Ed was a 5-handicap golfer with a passion for the golf swing. At least once a week he came to the office with a new "breakthrough"—a new way to hold the left hand, a new way to transfer weight, a new way to follow through. He was committed to teaching me the game, which I had played only sporadically as a teen-ager. His instruction was often confusing because things he taught me one day were often contradicted by his gestalt later in the week. On our occasional golf outings I would struggle around the course while Ed often hit two balls to hone the precision of his game. His commitment to the game was unquestioned.

On one very hot Washington day in 1961, the humidity was nearly 100%. At the 15th tee, I began to feel sweaty and light-headed with aching pressure in my upper chest. I immediately recognized these symptoms as classical for a heart attack. Not wanting to seem too hysterical, I described my symptoms to Ed, assuming he would share my concern and rush me to medical care. He pondered momentarily and then suggested that I lie down on a grassy knoll near the tee while he played through. He promised to come back for me after he finished the 18th hole. With great anxiety and nearly-continuous monitoring of my rapid radial pulse, I watched several groups of golfers tee off, observing me quizzically.

Ed did eventually come back in a golf cart. We drove to my V.A. laboratory where he performed an electrocardiogram which was completely normal. I was free of symptoms. The episode was deemed to be a mild case of heat stroke. Ed seldom veered from his planned task, but his judgment was impeccable. Despite my anxiety, he knew that nothing was seriously wrong. Good physicians can usually distinguish between functional disorders and real disease.

My research work during the first year of fellowship was directed to studying the effect of various new antihypertensive drugs on the circulation. What mediated the fall in blood pressure? Was it a decrease in force of contraction of the heart or was it relaxation of the arteries that determined the resistance to flow? Were arteries to some organs affected more than arteries to other organs? After all, the total resistance to blood flow, which accounts for the blood pressure, is composed of parallel resistances throughout the body that determine the blood flow to individual organs.

I became interested in assessing blood flow to individual organs, such as the kidney and liver, in an attempt to characterize the regional effect of hypertension and of drugs aimed at reducing blood pressure.

Erectile dysfunction circa 1960

My clinical work during that first fellowship year consisted of treating veterans in a hypertension clinic at the V.A. Hospital in Washington,

D.C. I was stunned at the frequency and severity of hypertension in that population, many of whom were African Americans. Our drug therapy was primitive on the basis of current standards, but we had drugs which, if given in adequate doses, could control blood pressure in most patients. Side effects of therapy, however, were considerable. The most troublesome to our male population was impotence, and most of the drugs that we used in those days were notorious for producing impotence. Erectile dysfunction, or E.D., was not a household word as it is today. Therefore, discussions of impotence were held behind closed doors after the nurse had been dismissed, and were mostly whispered confidences between the patient and the male doctor.

Knowing that we had no effective therapy to counter the impotence-generating side effect of the drugs, and no drugs that were effective in severe hypertension without causing impotence, I fell back on an old trick I had learned during my internship. Placebos, or sugar pills, can be remarkably effective in individuals with symptoms that are difficult to document. After one of my confidential encounters with a young black man who was distraught about his impotence, I told him, "I have a pill that may help you."

We maintained a small cabinet in the clinic with medications that were being used in certain trials. In the cabinet was a bottle of pink placebo tablets that had been used as a match for an active drug that we had previously studied. I carefully counted out 10 of these pills and placed them into a bottle on which I pasted a small label with the name, Hard A. The name was a last minute decision because I realized that I had to have a label on the pill bottle. I gave it to the patient and told him to take one prior to having sex.

Such deception with patients is unacceptable today, but in the 1960s there were few rules and regulations controlling the relationship between doctors and patients. There was no investigational review board, whose role today is to evaluate the ethics of any research effort. There was no consent form that would have required me to inform the patient that I might be giving him a placebo rather than an active drug. There was only the trust between the patient and the physician. In this instance, I realized I was violating that trust in the interest of relieving the patient of a troublesome symptom. Or perhaps I was relieving myself of the frustration of not having a solution to the patient's legitimate problem.

What I had failed to appreciate in providing the pink placebos was that all of our clinic patients sat in the waiting room sharing notes. Their weekly or biweekly visits to the clinic were often the high point of their social lives. They shared their experiences, their blood pressures, their side effects, and their medication experience. My patient not only found the pink pill remarkably effective, but also shared that information with all of his fellow patients, most of whom asked for the pink pill on subsequent visits. I realized I had created a serious problem, in part because my big bottle of pink pills was quickly running out.

I unsuccessfully queried the pharmacy and contacted several pharmaceutical companies to see whether anyone could provide us with a new supply of pink placebos. I did, however, find a source of yellow placebos and obtained a quantity adequate to supply the clinic for a number of months. Since they appeared so different from the other pills, I gave them a new name, Hard B. It was predictable, of course, that patients who believed in the pink pills would find the yellow pills less effective. Over the following months, I had to inform all the patients that we could no longer obtain the pink pills and they were limited to the Hard B medication in the yellow pills. The fascination for the placebo gradually waned.

This experience did not imply that the impotence was not genuine, not a side-effect of the drugs we used. Suggestion and confidence can sometimes over-ride functional disorders temporarily. But the disorder always returns. Impotence was a problem that could not be treated long-term with a placebo.

But there was hope on the horizon, unfortunately a more distant horizon than it needed to be. A pharmaceutical company had developed a new class of drug to lower blood pressure. They asked us if we would be willing to study its effects in a small group of hypertensive patients.

I recruited a dozen patients who were willing to try the new pill. As is always the case in such early trials, we had a long list of potential side effects , which we disclosed to the volunteers after they started taking the drug. Several men reported, smilingly, that they had noticed quite unexpected "hard-ons". I tossed this off as a form of sexual boasting un-related to the drug. One of our volunteers, however, was in the hospital for another reason when we initiated therapy with the new drug. On the third day of drug treatment, the aghast floor nurses found him next to his bed in the large patient ward masturbating. This was unusual enough to notice! Unfortunately, the drug was not very effective in lowering blood pressure and it had some other rather unpleasant side effects. The company, oblivious to our suggestion that they drug might have value as a sexual stimulant, discontinued its evaluation.

What we did not realize at the time, but became apparent years later, was that this drug was the first example of a new pharmacologic mecha-nism—inhibition of the body's rapid inactivation of cyclic GMP. Cyclic GMP is a normal product of cellular metabolism. It has a powerful re-laxing effect on small arteries, but its action is short-lived because of the body's rapid degradation of cyclic GMP. Relaxation of the small arteries in the penis is a prerequisite for an erection. Sexual stimulation normal-ly activates enough cyclic GMP to produce a sustained erection, despite its rapid rate of degradation. The anti-hypertensive drugs available at the time all reduced the amount of cyclic GMP produced.

The drug we had tested was the first agent that specifically inhibited the degradation of cyclic GMP in the penile arteries. By prolonging the action of cyclic GMP secreted in response to sexual stimulation, it led to an erection. It would be 40 years before Viagra, a drug with a sim-ilar mechanism of action, would reach the marketplace as a treatment for impotence. Had we recognized the potential value of this unwanted side-effect in the 1960s the management of E.D. might have been ad-vanced by many years.

Taking advantage of unwanted drug side-effects led to another "breakthrough" in our pharmacologic studies. We were provided with a new study drug identified by a research number. Animal studies showed it to be a powerful antihypertensive agent. We administered it to a series of volunteers, many of whom came back with unusual new hair growth, often in most bizarre locations such as their hands. The hair was atypical, more like fur than hair, and it was clearly unwanted. It was a side effect that limited the use of the drug, especially in women, but a dermatology colleague of mine was fascinated. He put it into an ointment, patented the product, and minoxidil became a successful agent to stimulate hair growth. The mechanism of that hair growth stimulation is as mysterious today as it was when we made the observation in the 1960s.

The kidney and hypertension

Since my research interest was in factors that raised blood pressure I became interested in the circulation of blood to the kidney. Renin is a substance secreted by the kidney and stored in granules that could be identified in the deep layers of the kidney. There was growing interest in the research community in the role of renin and its capacity to interact with a protein called angiotensinogen that is manufactured in the liver and normally circulates in the blood. Renin caused the breakdown of that protein into a potent artery constrictor called angiotensin. There were some in the research community who felt that hypertension was a complication of having too much renin in the blood, producing excess angiotensin that constricted the blood vessels and raised blood pressure. If that renin were coming from the kidney (which is the only place thought at that time to produce renin), then maybe the kidney was the cause of hypertension (Figure I- 4).

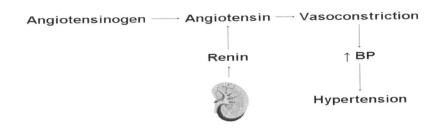

Figure I – 4
The kidney influences vascular resistance by its secretion of a hormone called renin. Renin in circulating blood leads to the production of angiotensinogen, a protein normally produced by the liver.

The hypothesis was that the kidney would release if the kidney blood flow was reduced. The biologic explanation for this reaction was that low blood flow, perhaps caused by a narrowing in the artery to a kidney, could be interpreted by the body to mean that the blood pressure had fallen. The body's response was therefore to secrete excess renin to raise blood pressure. This misinterpretation by the body, leading to an inappropriate response, could result in an unwanted rise in blood pressure. The design of the body had been misguided. Could this high renin hypertension account at least in part for the frequency of hypertension and the increased risk of heart attacks and strokes?

The renin system developed historically as humans evolved from fish and left the safety of salt water. A mechanism had to be available to conserve salt and respond to dehydration. The renin system provided a means for the kidney to detect a loss of volume and respond with the secretion of renin, which conserves salt and raises blood pressure. An overactive renin system might protect individuals from dehydration or blood loss and thus convey a potential survival advantage. On the other hand, long-term adverse consequences of an inappropriate renin-induced rise in blood pressure might shorten life. But these complications usually occur after the child-bearing years and would not therefore be expected to result in the evolutionary loss of the renin-protective mechanism.

A fortuitous clinical experience emphasized to me the complexity of the blood pressure control mechanisms. I was called to see Roger Pointer, a 43-year-old man who had been admitted to the hospital with a blood pressure of 210/140 mmHg, an elevation that could lead to catastrophic consequences such as brain hemorrhage. He had no prior history of hypertension, and this led to the concern that something acute had happened to his kidney blood flow, possibly precipitating the secretion of excess renin. He was treated acutely with a potent medication to lower his blood pressure, and his pressure fell precipitously to what the doctors considered a dangerously low level. Indeed, he appeared to be in shock, which will be discussed more thoroughly in the next chapter. The doctors were perplexed. This shock state led us to initiate a rapid infusion of intravenous fluids. His blood pressure stabilized at normal levels and the hypertension never reappeared.

After Roger stabilized, we carried out studies to explore his response to various stresses. This included plunging his hand into ice-water, a well-known stimulus to blood pressure elevation, and infusion of drugs to activate the sympathetic nervous system, which also raises blood pressure. On each occasion his blood pressure rose far more than normally anticipated, suggesting that his arteries had constricted to an unusual degree in response to these stresses. It was this constriction that was raising his blood pressure. His body had responded in exaggerated fashion to a message—probably a low blood volume in the circulation—transmitted in his sympathetic nervous system. A drop in blood flow (cardiac output) because of diminished circulating blood volume normally induce modest signals from the kidney and other tissues that instruct the arteries to constrict and prevent blood pressure from falling. In this patient the reflex response was overzealous and the blood pressure actually rose to dangerous levels.

Over the next few months I was called to see four other patients who presented with the same acute form of hypertension, and each of them also demonstrated this vascular hyper-responsiveness. I published these observations in the *New England Journal of Medicine* as a new clinical syndrome, paroxysmal hypertension related to volume depletion and effectively treated with volume expansion.

Tribal medicine

The dynamics of blood pressure control had never been more obvious to me.

I was beginning to think I understood blood pressure control mechanisms until I was confronted with a remarkably unusual patient. Gloria Banks was referred to my clinic by a local practitioner who was uncertain how to treat her blood pressure. She was a 25-year-old Native American woman who until a month before had been living on a reservation. She had moved to the city and was now living with a slightly older woman friend who had known her on the reservation. The woman asked to talk to me before I went into the examination room to see the patient. Gloria, she explained to me, had been given a hex of death by a medicine man and ostracized from the reservation. I never asked what she had done, but it wasn't hard to imagine. The whole idea seemed laughable, but I kept my composure and entered the room.

Gloria was a beautiful young woman with long black hair and sculpted features. She sat somberly in a chair and did not look up when I entered. The note from the doctor referred only to marked lability (constant change) of blood pressure that made it difficult to know what her true blood pressure was. Such lability is not uncommon and often takes the form of what is called "White Coat" hypertension, a dramatic rise of pressure in the presence of a doctor.

Gloria was non-communicative. I could not engage her in conversation. I asked her about the hex, and her only response suggested resignation. She apparently accepted that she was going to die. I couldn't get her interested in her blood pressure, which on several different readings in my office was ranged from 118/78 mm Hg, which is entirely normal, to 190/110 mmHg, which is extremely high. She didn't look any different when her blood pressure was very high, and her heart rate barely changed. I left the room and asked a nurse to come in every few minutes to measure the pressure in my absence. The nurse also found widely divergent readings.

The mystery of her wild fluctuations of pressure intrigued me. We needed to document it. I asked her to come into my laboratory for testing. As with everything else, she complied with no emotion.

I realized that we were dealing with cuff blood pressure readings, not the true pressure in the arteries. With her permission I placed a needle into the artery at her elbow crease and recorded pressures directly with a pressure sensor and a recorder. We could now accurately monitor pressure continuously with each heart beat to determine its fluctuation. The recordings were the most dramatic I have ever seen. She would begin with normal blood pressure of about 120/80 mmHg, then the pressure would rise dramatically to levels of nearly 200 mmHg. It would reside there for a minute or two and then fall gradually back to 120/80 mmHg. Nothing else seemed to change. These cycles would repeat themselves every few minutes without warning.

What was driving these short-lived episodes of pressure rise?

It had to be the brain, I theorized. Something about the hex had stimulated her brain to drive episodic blood pressure rises. This must be through the sympathetic nervous system, I reasoned. I could think of no way to prove the mechanism, but I asked her to collect her urine for a day so we could measure products of excessive secretion of sympathetic hormones, a condition called pheochromocytoma that can cause acute rises in blood pressure. The urine test was negative.

I prescribed a medication that was known to reduce the brain's sympathetic nerve discharge. I asked her to return in two weeks to observe the effect of the drug. As usual, she was little interested in the problem or in the treatment.

Her friend brought her back to the clinic in two weeks. She was still non-communicative and apparently resigned to her fate. I suspected she had not taken the medication. Her fluctuating blood pressure was again confirmed. That was the last time I saw her. She did not appear for her next visit. My nurse tried to reach her but there was no telephone contact in her record. Several months later a terse message was sent to the clinic. Gloria would not be coming back to clinic. She had died suddenly.

Voodoo death has been the subject of a number of scholarly reports that have collected cases, usually from Native American tribes. The mechanism of such events, other than the simple view that it is a response to fear, has never been clarified. It could be similar to a condition more recently recognized by cardiologists as the "Broken Heart Syndrome" or stress cardiomyopathy. In this condition, an extreme life stress, such as the loss of a loved one, leads to a sudden loss of heart muscle function, usually in the front wall of the heart. Not only does the heart pump fail but a lethal rhythm disturbance may occur. The name Takotsubo has been attached to the condition, because the stressed heart takes on the shape of a Japanese fishing pot for trapping octopus—a takotsubo.

All of these experiences emphasize the relationship between the brain and the cardiovascular system. Whether it's the effect of a placebo on impotence, the effect of anxiety on blood pressure, or the devastating effect of emotion on heart function or heart rhythm, these powerful forces are poorly understood. Whenever I think I am getting close to understanding the intricacies of cardiovascular disease, I recall Gloria and recognize how much we still have to learn.

But my interest at the time was Sam Farber, not the mystical experience of Gloria Banks. I was focused on learning what caused the sustained increase in blood pressure experienced by Sam and others who were classified as having essential hypertension. The most popular theory at the time was that the kidney was the culprit. Possibly, it was thought the kidney might be inappropriately secreting excess renin, which would raise the blood pressure. Perhaps renin secretion was increased when kidney blood flow fell, so maybe a reduction in kidney blood was the cause of hypertension.

Measuring blood flow to the kidney

To explore the relationship between blood flow to the kidney and hypertension, I realized that we needed a method for measuring blood flow. Dye-dilution techniques were in widespread use in the 1960s for measuring the amount of blood pumped by the heart. Early physiologists had invented the technique. A known quantity of a dye is injected rapidly into the blood flowing into the heart from the veins. The dye is diluted and mixed in its passage through the heart so that its concentration can be measured in an artery on the outflow side of the heart (Figure I-5).

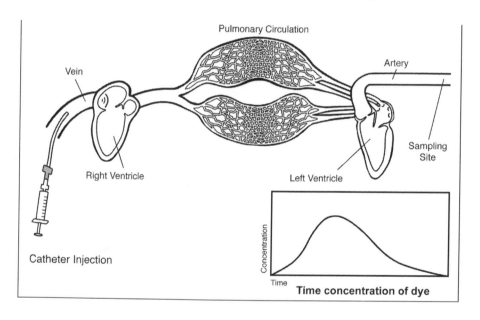

Figure I-5

Diagram of the dye dilution technique to calculate the amount of blood pumped by the heart (the cardiac output). A known quantity of dye is injected in a vein returning to the right ventricle. This dye is diluted and mixed in the blood flowing through the heart. Sampling the dye concentration in the blood in an artery, after it has traversed the right ventricle, the lungs and the left heart, allows the calculation of the amount of blood that flowed and diluted the dye during that time interval

By measuring the concentration of the dye in the artery (a dye curve) it is possible to calculate the amount of blood that passed through the heart in a given time and thus calculate the cardiac output over that interval. The accuracy of this technique for measuring cardiac output had been validated repeatedly in animals and in humans.

I thought that this dye-dilution technique could be applied to the kidney as well. It should be relatively easy, I reasoned, to thread thin plastic catheters under X-ray guidance from an artery and vein in the groin (femoral vessels) up to the renal (kidney) artery and renal vein. If we injected a known quantity of dye into the artery to the kidney, and sampled the concentration of dye in the vein leading from the kidney, we should be able to calculate the flow of blood through the kidney in a given period of time, just as we did across the heart to measure cardiac output (Figure I-5).

The V.A. Hospital had no cardiac catheterization laboratory, where such so-called invasive procedures would normally be performed, because they had no cardiologists. I had asked the Chief of Medicine in the early 1960s when I had arrived at the V.A. Hospital why they did not have a cardiologist on staff. He had responded that there were not enough cardiac patients to justify such a specialist. How bizarre that seems in today's world of specialization and the epidemic of cardiac disease.

In the absence of a cardiologist, I commandeered a small laboratory on an upper floor that had a radiographic (X-ray) table and a fluoroscopic unit for visualization. I found that catheterization of the kidney artery and vein was a simple procedure under fluoroscopy as long as one properly formed a curve on the end of these catheters before inserting them over a guide wire into the femoral vessels. I became adept at forming the curves, which was accomplished in hot water, and in threading the sterilized catheters into their proper place. The patients agreed to the procedure and suffered little discomfort.

We were now invading the kidney, an organ over which I had no authority. I was not a kidney specialist. I had no advanced training in kidney diseases. Fortunately, we had a new chief of nephrology at the V.A. Hospital. He was a physician from Yugoslavia, Ervin Gombos, who had trained at New York University with mentors who were well known to be skeptical of efforts to use drugs to lower blood pressure.

Despite our fundamental conceptual disagreement, Erv and I had become friends. Syma and I socialized with Erv and his wife, Adrienne.

She was a pianist, as was Syma. I was still devoted to my violin in those days, and Syma and I had tried to play Mozart sonatas together with disastrous results. We knew each other too well to tolerate our individual deficiencies. Had we continued that effort, our marriage would likely have been doomed. Perhaps our 62 years together can be attributed in part to the fact that we never again tried to play duets.

I turned instead to Adrienne, who was delighted to have weekly duet sessions with me. The four of us even planned a week's holiday together in Jamaica, where we rented adjoining cottages on a private beach staffed by a beach boy and housekeepers who prepared our meals. The week was memorable, not only because of the friendship, the environment, the tranquility and the romantic time Syma and I spent together without the burden of my research, but because it was where I grew my beard. What began as a week-long holiday from shaving became a life-long facial growth which has never left my chin, even as it changed over the years from black to gray.

Erv agreed to work with me on the measurement of kidney blood flow and to review with me the X-rays we took of the arteries to the kidney outlined by dye injected into the catheter in the renal artery. We published these results in 1965. We later studied kidney blood flow in a wide range of clinical conditions, including hypertension, to define not only the total blood flow to the kidney but even the distribution of blood flow between the superficial blood vessels in the kidney, which flow very quickly, and the deeper levels of the kidney, which flow more slowly.

We also collected blood from the renal vein to measure the concentration of angiotensin as a guide to the kidney's production of that hormone. Measurement of angiotensin was complicated in those days. No chemical assay had yet been developed, so it was necessary to use a bioassay. Bioassays measure the effect of a substance on a tissue as a guide to its concentration. For that purpose you need a tissue that responds uniquely to the substance you want to identify, and a method for measuring that response. It had previously been shown that angiotensin exerts a unique pattern of effect on the muscle of stomach, intestine and colon. No other substance had such a pattern of response—constricting the smooth muscle of some organs and not of others. Therefore, to perform the assay, we established a tissue bath in which strips of rat stomach, intestine, and colon were attached to devices to measure their contraction and mounted into a chamber where they were bathed with a warm salt solution. Blood sampled from the renal vein was then added to the bathing salt solution. The behavior of the strips of rat tissue told us how much angiotensin was in the renal vein blood. We could then calculate the angiotensin production from the kidney and its relationship to blood flow.

Do I specialize in the kidney or the heart?

This work was going well in the late 1960s and we were reporting our observations in medical meetings and in medical journals. I was an active member of two new societies, the American Society of Nephrology and the International Society of Nephrology which were dedicated to study of the kidney. But I became growingly aware that the kidney was behaving passively, responding to the blood flow provided to it by the heart. Yes, the kidney received a disproportionate amount of that blood flow, about 20% of cardiac output, a lot for a couple of small organs. But the reason for the blood flow was to cleanse the body of wastes, not to nourish the organ or influence its health. It was the heart that nourished all the organs. The heart was the master organ.

All clinical research depends upon a willing patient and a willing referring doctor. Since I spent much of my time on the wards of the V.A. Hospital helping residents and senior staff manage their sick patients, I earned the trust of most of these referring physicians. They shared with me cases that they thought might be of interest to my research program.

I was called one day to see a 49-year-old man, Stanley Williams, who was admitted with untreated severe hypertension and was complaining of shortness of breath. The physicians caring for him could find no evidence of heart failure, which would be the usual reason for shortness of breath in a hypertensive patient, but they had begun drug therapy and his blood pressure had not responded very well. I suggested that we bring him to the laboratory to check his renal blood flow and visualize the arteries to his kidneys, since blockage of an artery to the kidney is a powerful stimulus to the release of angiotensin which might be raising his blood pressure. No drugs were available at that time to block the effects of angiotensin, as compared to today when ACE inhibitors (angiotensin converting enzyme inhibitors), angiotensin receptor blockers and the new direct renin inhibitors have become standard therapy for hypertension. But we were occasionally operating on obstructed renal arteries to restore blood flow and reduce the stimulus for renin release.

Heart failure was not easily diagnosed in those days. The chest x-ray was the preferred tool. One looked for an enlarged cardiac silhouette and evidence for increased markings in the lung fields suggesting accumulated fluid. Although Mr. Williams' x-ray showed what we interpreted as a slightly enlarged left ventricle—the pumping chamber of his heart—the overall cardiac silhouette was not enlarged and the lung fields appeared normal. The veins in the neck were also usually engorged in heart failure because of the back-up of fluid behind the heart and the ankles are often swollen. Mr. Williams exhibited neither of these signs.

Since he complained of shortness of breath without a good explanation, it occurred to me that perhaps while studying the kidney we might also be able to thread the catheter all the way up the aorta and through the aortic valve into the left ventricle of the heart, where we could directly measure the pressure in the left ventricle as a possible cause of his shortness of breath (Figure I-6).

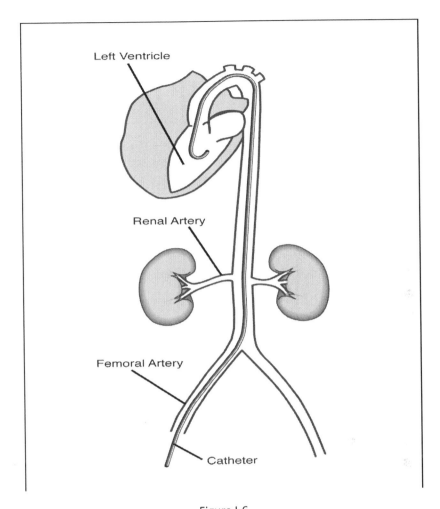

Figure I-6

Diagram of a catheter passed from the femoral artery in the groin, up the aorta, past the kidneys and through the aortic valve into the left ventricle of the heart

Such retrograde catheterization of the left ventricle was indeed being performed in some cardiac catheterization laboratories, usually to evaluate the health of the aortic valve. I decided that this should be a simple enough procedure. I fashioned a catheter with a tear-drop-shaped loop on the end, which I thought would allow it to more easily traverse the aortic valve and plunk into the left ventricle. I could watch the tip of the catheter under fluoroscopy as I pushed it up the aorta from the groin.

After completing the study of the kidney with an especially long catheter, I pushed the catheter further up the aorta and watched as the teardrop knuckle of the curve reached the aortic valve and then, with a slight additional push, entered the left ventricle. Nothing untoward happened except for a few ventricular premature beats (electrical impulses generated when the catheter tickled the inner lining of the left ventricle).

When the catheter was attached to our pressure transducer it was clear we were recording left ventricular pressures. The pressure in this patient's left ventricle was remarkably abnormal. When heart failure is present, the pressure in the left ventricle during diastole—before the next contraction—is elevated. It is that elevated pressure in the left ventricle, a manifestation of inadequate emptying of the heart, which is transmitted back to the lung that accounts for shortness of breath. A normal left ventricular diastolic pressure is less than 12 mmHg. This patient's pressure was 30 mmHg, thus confirming the diagnosis of heart failure even though the patient presented with no signs of heart failure. We had indeed shown that heart failure could be diagnosed in the absence of clinical signs.

The procedure of entering the left ventricle was so simple that after 10 or 12 additional experiences in the catheterization laboratory I concluded that we should be able to do the procedure without fluoroscopy or X-ray. This could make the procedure suitable for bedside studies in patients that were deemed in those days to be too sick to go to the catheterization laboratory.

We then did a few cases in the catheterization laboratory without turning on the fluoroscope. In each instance I advanced a catheter until the electrocardiographic monitor identified one or two extra beats indicating that the catheter had slipped into the left ventricle. In each instance we successfully recorded left ventricular pressure without complications.

We were ready to embark on a much more exciting research enterprise. The function of the heart is a critical factor in determining blood pressure and in supporting life. In Sam Farber's case, the failure of healthy interaction between the heart and the arteries must have killed him.

We now had a tool that could allow us to monitor the function of the pumping chamber of the heart in acutely ill patients. U.S. Catheter, the company that at that time marketed vascular catheters to health care providers, even listed my self-designed curved catheter in their catalogue (without any agreement with me) as the Cohn Catheter for LV pressure measurement. I doubt if any were ever sold. We used our own. A treasure trove of new insights awaited us.

I have often referred back to that first experience, in 1970, when we recorded left ventricular pressure and diagnosed heart failure, as the moment when I became a cardiologist. But I became a different kind of cardiologist than most of those who practiced at the time. Since I entered the heart from the arteries, I was acutely aware of the importance of the circulation in impacting on the heart. It is their integration that controls the flow of blood to tissues, which is the main role of the heart's function.

Four years later I was recruited to the University of Minnesota to become chief of cardiology. (They apparently viewed me as a cardiologist.) I had for some years been acquainted with a well-known Minnesota cardiac surgeon, Rich Lillehei, who was fond of belittling cardiologists as "tinkerers". He accused them of viewing the heart as a "music box" rather than as a pumping organ. Cardiology rounds in Minnesota and elsewhere in those days often involved a patient lying on a stretcher with a conference leader holding a stethoscope to the patient's chest. Everyone in the audience listened with their own stethoscope connected to an electronic system that amplified the sounds received by the stethoscope on the patient's chest. The gamesmanship involved determining who could hear a specific murmur. My surgical colleague viewed this exercise as a form of autoeroticism that was not dedicated to helping the patient. He was a doer, not a listener. He fixed things. Cardiologists just listened and talked.

One of my first acts in Minnesota was to change the name of our medical school division from "Cardiology" to "Cardiovascular", to emphasize that the heart and blood vessels could not be separated. Listening to the heart was not discouraged, but it became growingly clear that seeing, feeling, and measuring were equally important skills to hone, and newer technologies had made listening less critical. Treatments could be developed if we understood the problem, and these treatments need not be surgical. Cardiologists had the opportunity to do more than listen. They had access to tools that could greatly enhance their evaluation of patients, and they had the potential for innovative drug therapy that could dramatically change the course of patients with cardiovascular disease.

Physicians still display their stethoscopes, often wrapped casually around their necks, as a symbol of their professional competence. But the stethoscope is largely vestigial. It serves as a display of hands-on involvement with patients but provides relatively modest insight into the heart and its function.

My "music box" era had ended when I catheterized the left ventricle. The University of Minnesota would be different. We would not sit around fiddling with our stethoscopes. We would view, study and treat the heart as a component of a complex system that was the overall determinant of cardiovascular health. Our goal, similar to my surgical colleague's but with far more diversified tools, was to make the patient better without necessarily cutting open his or her chest.

CHAPTER II
Shock

Sam Farber died of a clinical condition called "shock". It is the most dramatic example of the complex cardiovascular system gone awry. Without effective treatment it is almost always lethal within hours.

When I arrived at the V.A. Hospital as a research fellow in 1960, shock was a major clinical problem. Every medical ward had one or two patients in shock at any given time. I became interested in shock, not only to try to understand how I might better have treated Sam Farber, but because shock represented a condition the opposite of hypertension.

In hypertension, the blood pressure is too high. This elevated pressure is thought to exert long-term adverse effects on the heart and blood vessels. In shock the blood pressure is too low, and this low blood pressure was thought to impair blood flow to critical organs that were necessary for survival. Blood pressure was thought to be key in both cases—too high in hypertension, and too low in shock. That was why we had treated Sam when he was in shock with drugs designed to raise blood pressure.

The low blood pressure of shock was detected by the same technique as the high blood pressure of hypertension. A cuff was wrapped on the upper arm and pressurized with air. As the cuff was deflated, sounds are generated by blood flow in the artery as the cuff pressure falls below the arterial systolic (top number) pressure. A stethoscope amplifies these sounds. The systolic pressure is assumed to be the pressure in the cuff when the first sound is heard during cuff deflation.

The diagnosis of shock was made when that pressure was abnormally low (usually less than 90mmHg) especially when accompanied by signs of inadequate circulation, including cool, clammy skin; reduced urine output (kidney blood flow); and somnolence or confusion (brain blood flow). The standard treatment was to infuse a drug which constricted the blood vessels thus raising the blood pressure.

What a paradox! Here we were trying to lower blood pressure in hypertension by relaxing constricted arteries without understanding the reason for their constriction. And now we were infusing drugs in shock to constrict the arteries without understanding if or why they had dilated. I was struck by the irrationality of the therapeutic approach. It was all aimed at maintaining blood pressure within some so-called normal range. And all of this was based on a broad assumption that the blood pressure cuff provided an accurate assessment of the true pressure in the artery.

Why is blood pressure low?

In 1963 I discussed the knowledge gap with my mentor, Ed Freis, and he agreed that a study of the circulation in such patients could be very informative. How could we better treat the condition if we didn't understand what was wrong? Simply knowing the blood pressure is too low provides little insight into this complex system. It does not tell us whether the heart is not pumping enough blood, or if the arteries are too relaxed to support blood pressure.

The problem was that these patients were too sick to move to a laboratory where we had all the necessary equipment to study them properly. Critically ill patients at that time were not in intensive care units because such units had yet to be developed. The patients were maintained on open wards or in semi-private rooms. We had to bring the laboratory to the patient. And that would not be easy, because the patient rooms were cramped, and sick patients were surrounded by equipment and staff that would make it particularly difficult to bring in our own equipment and personnel.

I liberated an unused rolling cart from a remote corridor, salvaged an old recorder that would allow us to document pressures and flows, took some pressure transducers, a blood pump and a densitometer (a device that allowed us to perform dye dilution studies) from our hemodynamic study laboratory, and acquired an array of sterilized catheters and needles. The problem with the old recorder (I had no funds for a new one) was that I had to constantly readjust the tiny mirrors that were critical to focus the signals onto photographic recording paper. Moving the cart from my lab to the various hospital wards often displaced the mirrors. I accepted this inconvenience as part of the research experience.

We were almost ready to embark on our mission to characterize the heart and circulatory function in patients with shock. I was convinced that a better understanding of the circulatory abnormalities would lead to far more rational and effective therapy. But we were missing one key element. I needed a technician to help with the mobile cart and the procedures. This was not a one-person activity, and the young physicians who often worked with me did not have the time or technical skill to serve. The V.A. agreed to pay for a technician and I started recruiting. I knew I would have to train whoever I hired, because few people had been trained to do the kind of clinical research work I was undertaking. I decided a college biology graduate might be ideal, especially if the person was bright, enthusiastic and anxious to learn. I placed an ad in the Washington Post for a junior scientist.

One of the first applicants seemed perfect. Claire had just graduated from a local Catholic college with outstanding grades in science. She was personable and enthusiastic. All her older siblings were in health care and she was anxious to learn—as well as anxious to be efficient and to please. She joined the team and I spent a week training her on all the equipment, methods and procedures we would be using. She was a quick study. Her manual dexterity was excellent. Soon, she and I were both confident she was ready for action. I spread the word on the medical wards that we were interested in studying patients in shock. I did not have a long wait.

Edward Cronin was a 66-year-old man who had been admitted several days before with pneumonia, but despite antibiotics his condition had deteriorated. During the night his blood pressure had begun to fall. The green curtains were drawn around his bed in the large open ward and I parted them. He appeared unconscious and was sweating profusely. I attempted to introduce myself. "Mr. Cronin," I said close to his ear. But he did not respond. A catheter drainage tube was traversing from beneath the sheet into a bag hanging on the bed. I noticed that he had no urine output. A blood pressure cuff encircled his right upper arm and was attached to a wall manometer. An IV dripped at a steady rate into a vein in his left arm. I read the handwritten label on the bottle: Levophed. It was the same drug we had administered to Sam Farber some years before when his blood pressure had fallen.

Levophed is the trade name for norepinephrine, a potent hormone secreted by nerve endings in the blood vessels and the heart to constrict the blood vessels and stimulate the heart to contract more forcefully. It is also known as noradrenalin, a cousin of adrenalin, which is secreted by the adrenal gland in response to stress – the well-known "adrenalin rush" that raises blood pressure and causes heart palpitations. Its use in patients with shock was aimed at supporting a falling blood pressure to keep the vital organs adequately nourished by blood. Unfortunately, the rise in pressure was accompanied by artery constriction that often impeded an increase in blood flow. Also, the rise in pressure added a further burden to the heart, which may already be suffering from inadequate nutrition to meet its metabolic work needs. So, although Levophed was often used as the first line of defense in patients with low blood pressure and shock, it rarely was life-saving. Nearly everyone who developed shock without a correctable cause died with or without Levophed.

A nurse slipped in to check the IV drip and re-measure blood pressure. She pumped up the cuff on the arm and listened with her stethoscope as the cuff pressure fell, sadly shaking her head. "No sounds," she said, the first sign that she acknowledged my presence. "But I can feel a weak pulse below 120." She made a notation on the clipboard at the side of the bed: "BP 120 (palpatory)." She left the drip unchanged and departed for other duties.

Blood pressure as traditionally assessed doesn't actually measure pressure directly. It relies on two imperfect principles: 1) that the cuff around the arm, when inflated to a pressure above the pressure in the artery deep in the arm, will obstruct the artery; and 2) that when the artery opens because of deflation of the cuff (systolic pressure), flow in the artery will generate a sound that will be heard with each beat until the cuff pressure falls to a level at which the artery is no longer obstructed during any part of the heart beat (diastolic pressure). That was, and is, the standard method for measuring blood pressure in clinics and hospitals.

But nurses knew that in some sick patients the sounds were not audible. They relied instead on feeling the pulse at the wrist, which disappears when the cuff pressure is higher than the systolic pressure and should reappear when the cuff pressure falls below systolic pressure. Thus, "by palpation".

Sometimes you couldn't *feel* a pulse either. Under those circumstances the pressure was often recorded as "0", although no one truly thought that there was no pressure in the artery, especially if the patient was alive. Not much thought was given to why there were no sounds over the artery, or why the pulse could not be felt. It was merely a clinical observation dutifully transcribed in the record. It was assumed it was due to low pressure.

I was about to leave the bedside to call my team when a priest parted the curtain, prepared to give last rites. It subsequently became a ghoulish joke in the hospital: "It's a race as to who gets to the bedside first, the priest or Jay Cohn."

Edward Cronin's wife and two adult children were in the family waiting room. I introduced myself and explained the grave state of Edward's circulation. I told them how we planned to find a treatment to reverse his shock. They agreed to the procedure.

A study at the bedside

Squeezing our cart of equipment into the space near the bed—which was already surrounded by IV poles, blood pressure cuffs and an oxygen tank—was a feat. Nurses immediately took a dislike to our presence because we interfered with their access to the patient.

Two procedures were necessary: a tube would be introduced into a vein and threaded toward the heart for measurement of pressure, and for injections; a needle would be placed into an artery through which we could record pressure and sample blood. We usually tried to use the arm for these insertions. But sometimes, because pulses were too weak to guide our needles, we resorted to using the femoral artery, which was far easier to locate in the groin.

We chose the groin for Mr. Cronin because his pulse there was easily palpable. I worked on the femoral artery while Myron Luria, my junior colleague, dealt with placement of a plastic tube through a needle in an arm vein.

Placing a catheter or tube in the femoral artery involves inserting a needle into the groin at the site of the pulsation. When the needle enters the artery, a spurt of blood heralds its position and allows a fine guide wire to be passed through the needle. This guide wire maintains access for the subsequent insertion of a plastic tube, which is threaded over the guidewire.

Claire was prepared for the procedure. She was gowned and gloved for sterility, as were Myron and I. She handed me the needle and then the wire and the catheter. After completing the procedure I turned back to her for gauze pads to mop up the escaped blood.

She wasn't there.

My eyes darted around the room to find her. She was nowhere to be seen, until I glanced down. She had passed out. My training had covered all contingencies except the sight of blood. To her remarkable credit she recovered quickly and resumed her post, somewhat pale and sweaty. It was our first and last experience with research team loss of consciousness.

Once the transducer was attached to the arterial catheter, the recorder quickly identified a problem. The blood pressure, which was being supported by a Levophed drip at 120 mmHg based on the cuff measurement, was actually 180 mmHg when recorded directly from the artery. Edward was clearly being over-treated with Levophed.

Perhaps Sam Farber also hadn't need the Levophed we had given him seven years earlier. If Levophed had increased Sam's pressure to 180 mmHg, maybe that's why his heart failed and he died. Obviously, the cuff was not an adequate way to measure blood pressure in patients with shock. At that moment, the problem was not that Mr. Cronin's blood pressure was too low, but rather that his blood flow to the brain, kidney, and perhaps other organs was inadequate.

I vowed at that moment to devise an experiment to test the accuracy of cuff blood pressure measurements when blood flow was reduced. Three years later we published the results of that study in the *Journal of the American Medical Association*. When Levophed or noradrenalin was infused in a small dose into the artery supplying the arm, the constrictor effect of the drug reduced flow to that arm without changing blood pressure, which was not affected by the small local infusion of the drug. But the pulse in the radial artery at the wrist was weakened, and the cuff blood pressure could not be recorded because the sounds over the artery disappeared.

The sounds heard through the stethoscope are dependent on adequate blood flow when the cuff is deflated. When flow is reduced, even though pressure is high, the sounds disappear.

Pulsations felt over an artery are dependent on an entirely different set of conditions. When the heart pumps, the pulsation that we feel depends on compressing the artery with your fingers between pulsations. Try this: feel the pulse at your wrist on the thumb side. Notice the wave that strikes your finger which each beat. That's the pressure wave distending the artery. But what if the artery was a rigid steel tube instead of a flexible tube? You wouldn't feel the pulse because the pressure wave would not expand the tube. It was clear, then, that Levophed made the artery wall stiff and obscured the pulsation. Shock did the same thing. We had reproduced the problem that almost caused Edward Cronin's death, and may have contributed to Sam Farber's death.

We turned off Mr. Cronin's Levophed infusion and watched as his directly measured arterial pressure fell, settling at about 100 mmHg. We also watched the pressure recorded from the catheter which Myron had threaded from a vein in the arm into the right atrium of the heart. This is the heart chamber into which all the veins drain, and is the source of pressure to fill the pumping chamber. This pressure had started at five mmHg, a normal value when the Levophed was being infused, but fell to 0 mmHg as the Levophed effect waned. It was thus clear that the pumping chamber—the ventricle—was now under-filled. Mr. Cronin did not have adequate volume in his heart to pump enough blood.

We had also been busy measuring the output of the heart—the amount of blood pumped each minute. This method required injecting a dye into the right atrium and withdrawing blood from the femoral artery through a densitometer that detected the concentration of dye as it reached the femoral artery. This dye dilution technique told us that his cardiac output was very low, thus accounting for the inadequacy of blood flow to his vital organs.

Viewing his circulatory disturbance, Myron and I reached the same conclusion simultaneously.

"He needs more blood volume," we both said. And he needed it urgently!

Why would Mr. Cronin need extra volume in his circulation? He had not suffered from a hemorrhage, which is the usual cause of low blood volume. He had not become dehydrated because of insufficient water and fluids. He had been under observation in the hospital and was receiving intravenous fluids. None of his care providers suspected that he was volume depleted. In fact, they had thought that failure of his heart accounted for his shock.

But this was not heart failure. The low output from his heart was a direct consequence of not having enough blood in his heart to pump.

And it wasn't that he lacked red blood cells. He hadn't lost blood; he had lost plasma, the high protein fluid in which the red blood cells swim.

Dextran is a carbohydrate product with particle sizes similar to the protein in blood plasma. It is still used as a substitute for human plasma and is readily available on the shelf as a plasma volume expander. We attached a bottle to Mr. Cronin's IV tube and it dripped in rapidly. After 500 ccs, or about a pint, his right atrial pressure was still only two mmHg, and his blood pressure 105 mmHg. We hung up a second bottle and he began to respond. He stopped sweating and opened his eyes. Urine started dripping into the bag on his bed. His right atrial pressure was now six mmHg; his blood pressure 120/70 mmHg; and his cardiac output was nearly normal.

His shock was reversed.

Where oh where did it go?

Where had Mr. Cronin's plasma gone? Could it be that the stress hormone released by the sympathetic nervous system (and also infused in the form of Levophed) actually deplete plasma volume? Could stress, and the treatment we were using, be the causes of the inadequate blood volume?

I designed an experiment to test the hypothesis. Normal volunteers, who I always seemed able to recruit, were given infusions of noradrenalin (Levophed) and other related hormones normally released under stress. We monitored blood flow to the arm to assess the degree of arterial constriction. We monitored the tone of the veins which drain the blood from the arm. We also monitored the subject's plasma volume. This is done by injecting a known quantity of labeled albumin, which remains in the blood stream and is mixed with the plasma. The concentration level of this labeled albumin reveals the volume of plasma into which the label was injected.

The capillary is the business end of the arterial system. The capillaries have thin walls that transport nutrients from the blood stream to the tissues. These thin walls can also transport fluid. If the capillary pressure is low, fluid may be absorbed from the tissues into the capillaries, expanding plasma volume. If the capillary pressure is high, however, fluid may be transported out of the capillary, resulting in reduced plasma volume.

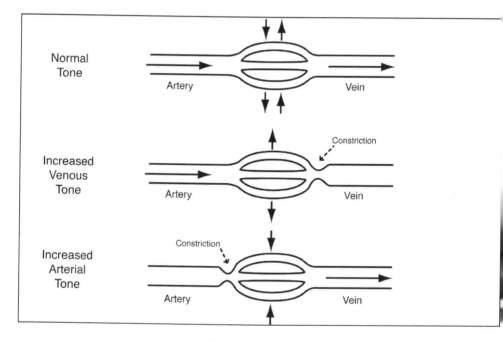

Figure II-1

Diagram of the control of capillary pressure. Under normal circumstances of arterial inflow pressure and venous outflow resistance, capillary pressure is maintained at a level at which there is a balance of forces (short arrows) controlling filtration of fluid out of the blood stream and back into the blood stream. When the veins are constricted the capillary pressure is increased and fluid leaves the circulation. When the small arteries are constricted capillary pressure is reduced and fluid is absorbed into the circulatory system.

The capillary pressure is determined by the balance between the resistance to flow from the arteries into the capillaries and the resistance to flow out of the capillaries into the veins (Figure II-1). I viewed it as a ratio of venous tone to arterial resistance. When the vein was constricted because of a high venous tone, blood would be backed up in the capillary and capillary pressure would be high. This would lead to leakage of fluid out of the capillary and a depletion of plasma volume. When the arterial resistance was high, flow into the capillary would be inhibited and the capillary pressure would fall. Under those circumstances, fluid would be absorbed from the tissues into the circulation and plasma volume would rise.

Our study of the volunteers confirmed the hypothesis. During infusion of noradrenalin (or Levophed) and its cousin hormones, the venous tone increased more than the arterial resistance. Capillary pressure must have risen (we couldn't actually measure it) because there was a striking depletion of plasma volume. The mechanism of Mr. Cronin's volume depletion, we concluded, had been an increase in capillary pressure induced by constriction of the veins that are exquisitely sensitive to stress hormones.

After the experience with Mr. Cronin, nurses were less critical of our presence at the bedside. Indeed, our remarkable success with this first patient resulted in frequent calls to minister to similarly ill patients. Many of these also exhibited evidence for unrecognized volume depletion, which responded to volume expansion with dextran.

The management of shock was forever changed at the V.A. Hospital and, as our publications became widely recognized, at other institutions around the world. I received annual Christmas cards from the Cronins. They apparently recognized how close Edward had come to not celebrating another Christmas.

Alcohol, the kidney and the liver

But my horizons were expanded when Sheldon, a senior medical resident, called me for advice about managing one of his patients, a cirrhotic with low blood pressure and no urine output.

Liver cirrhosis was a common disease at the V.A. Hospital. As I walked through the wards, the tell-tale signs were apparent in many beds: a mountain covered by a sheet and a small yellow face. The mountain, of course, was the abdomen distended with fluid (ascites). The yellow face was from jaundice caused by liver failure.

Cirrhotic patients were very different from the other patients I had been working with. Cirrhotics usually had a self-inflicted disease, and they knew it. They were often alone because their alcoholism had chased away spouses and family. They were often less motivated to fight their disease. I hadn't thought much about their circulatory systems because they were cared for by one of several V.A. gastroenterologists. I was interested in blood pressure, the kidney and the heart. I hadn't thought about the gastrointestinal circulation or the liver.

"Do you think he's in shock?" Sheldon asked about his cirrhotic patient.

Melvin Green was 47 years old. A construction worker who had consumed prodigious amounts of alcohol over the prior 10 years, Melvin had been divorced for four years and hadn't seen his two children since that time. This was his third hospitalization for jaundice and ascites, but things had obviously taken a turn for the worse. His kidneys had stopped functioning.

When I visited his bedside, Melvin was friendly and genial. I felt his abdomen, which was distended and taut from the ascites. I checked his blood pressure with a cuff on the arm. As reported by the resident, it was very low: 76/40 mmHg. I trusted the reading since Melvin's skin was warm and the sounds heard over the artery were strong.

This was not the kind of shock in which blood flow to the extremities is markedly reduced. In that kind of shock, brain blood flow is markedly reduced and patients are often unresponsive. Melvin was very lucid despite his low blood pressure. His brain was obviously well perfused with blood. In fact, it was well known that cirrhotics often have a high cardiac output, presumably from the shunting of blood somewhere in the circulation. So despite the low blood pressure and impaired kidney function, this wasn't shock.

Or was it?

The literature called this rather common complication of cirrhosis "hepatorenal syndrome". All the name implied was that there was some link between the liver and the kidney. No one really understood it, but the appearance of kidney failure in the cirrhotic usually was a terminal phase of the disease. There was no known treatment. The resident had asked me for advice about treatment and, in the process, had sparked an idea that maybe this was the same as shock—a decrease in organ blood flow, a hemodynamic problem.

That night I couldn't get Melvin out of my mind. If his kidneys were failing because of inadequate blood flow, it wasn't reflected by inadequate flow to the rest of his body. Maybe the pressure of the ascites had been having an adverse effect on his kidney blood flow. Maybe, although his cardiac output was not low, it was lower than it needed to be to nourish his kidneys. Maybe it was *something like shock*. If he was in shock, maybe we should acutely expand his blood volume.

The next morning, I again visited Melvin at his bedside. He was pleased to see me. Things hadn't changed. I proposed to him that we would put a catheter up a vein in his arm to determine the pressure of blood filling his heart. He agreed.

The pressure in the right atrium was zero and his blood pressure still 75/44 mmHg. He certainly needed volume expansion, I concluded. But fluid given to a cirrhotic tends to go right into his abdominal cavity in the form of ascites.

The solution, I decided, was to take out the ascites fluid and infuse it into his circulation.

Ascites is formed by plasma from circulating blood seeping through the blood vessel walls—usually in the intestine—and then accumulating in the abdominal cavity. It is a product of blood and, except for red blood cells, contains similar constituents as blood. I saw no reason why we couldn't put it back in the blood stream where it belonged. Melvin agreed without really understanding it.

The main thing was to keep the fluid sterile between its removal and reinfusion. I decided the best approach would be to put a needle into the abdomen to drain the fluid, and then attach the needle to tubing that would run directly into the venous catheter we had put in Melvin's arm.

The pressure in the abdomen, I reasoned, would probably drive the fluid into the vein. But I decided to assist the infusion with a roller pump we had in the laboratory. This pump compressed the tubing as it rolled, pumping the fluid forward. The pumping began slowly at first, to make certain nothing unexpected happened, and then more rapidly as it became apparent Melvin was tolerating it well.

It didn't take long to observe the response. After about one liter was infused Melvin's blood pressure had increased to 100/70 mmHg and he began to form prodigious quantities o urine. Melvin was pretty unemotional about the whole thing. Since he had a catheter in his bladder he didn't pay much attention to the copious flow of urine. But the nurses and residents did. We had done the impossible. We had cured hepatorenal syndrome!

But *cure* wasn't the right word. We had temporarily reversed the problem by expanding the blood volume, relieving the abdominal pressure and apparently increasing kidney blood flow. Melvin was delighted with his flat belly the next day. Quite predictably, however, when we removed the needle and discontinued the infusion the syndrome gradually recurred. The ascites began re-accumulating and the kidney function gradually declined.

This was not the same as the kind of shock in which treatment with volume expansion cured the problem. We weren't sure why the volume had become depleted in those earlier patients, and their problem was clearly reversible. These cirrhotic patients had a structural reason for their volume depletion. The liver was scarred and obstructing the blood flow that usually passed through its blood vessels with no resistance. It was like the capillaries in Figure II-1. The blood flow was obstructed in the veins, and capillary pressure rose behind the liver. The weeping of fluid out of the capillaries of the liver and intestine produced fluid in the abdomen and depleted the plasma volume. It was *almost* like shock—but volume expansion was only temporary because we couldn't reverse the cause.

To prove that low kidney blood flow was the problem, we next measured kidney blood flow in other patients with hepatorenal syndrome using our dye dilution method. As expected, the blood flow was very low, even though their cardiac output was high. Obviously, the arteries to the kidney were constricted. Could we infuse a drug directly into the artery that would dilate the arteries in that kidney and increase blood flow?

Would an increase in blood flow improve kidney function in a patient with hepatorenal syndrome?

A Rube Goldberg moment

To answer those questions I performed one of those experiments that led Michael Halberstam, a physician-newspaper columnist for the Washington Post, to describe me—in a column years later on how heretical thinking changes medicine—as doing strange but creative things to patients in order to improve their outcomes.

In the laboratory I threaded a catheter into the artery to the right kidney of a patient with hepatorenal syndrome and infused acetylcholine, a known arterial dilator. By infusing it directly into the kidney I could use a very low dose that would have no effect on the rest of the body. The kidney blood flow rose briskly, so I left the catheter in the artery and returned the patient to his bed where we continued a slow infusion for 24 hours. The patient's urine flow, presumably only from the right kidney, increased dramatically.

We now knew that hepatorenal syndrome was a shock-like state of the kidneys. The kidneys were being deprived of adequate blood flow, but the rest of the body was getting excess blood flow. We also knew that we could infuse a vasodilator directly into the kidney to increase its flow and restore urine production.

Could there be a simpler way to accomplish the same thing?

A drug company was exploring the effect of synthetic derivatives of vasopressin, a circulating hormone formed in the pituitary gland. It was also known as anti-diuretic hormone because its primary purpose was to instruct the kidney to retain water. This hormone was known to be a potent blood vessel constrictor, thus its other name, vasopressin. Vasopressin is composed of amino acids, and the drug company had investigated substitutions for the naturally occurring amino acids to alter its activity. They were excited about a compound in which phenylalanine and lysine had been substituted for the usual arginine in the molecule. It was now a *drug* and not a *hormone*, giving it an economic advantage. The drug was called PLV2, for phenylalanine-lysine vasopressin. In experimental animals, PLV2 constricted most arteries, but not those to the kidney. It appeared to be a *selective* constrictor.

I wondered if this experimental drug could accomplish the same redistribution of blood flow to the kidney as did our direct infusion of acetylcholine into the kidney. When we infused PLV2 in a group of patients with hepatorenal failure, the blood pressure rose—just as the company scientists had predicted—because it was a generalized constrictor of blood vessels. But the kidney blood flow rose, thus resulting in a redistribution of blood flow toward the kidney and a rise in urine output.

It was just what we were looking for, a drug that at least partially corrected the circulatory abnormality in advanced cirrhosis with hepatorenal syndrome. It quickly became apparent, however, that our quest was fruitless. The effect was maintained only as long as we infused the drug. Long-term infusion was impractical and would probably be accompanied by a waning of action or unwanted side effects. No drug was going to reverse the profound abnormality of the circulation in advanced liver disease. We could do heroic things to make the kidney produce urine, but we couldn't make the patient better. We were molesting them with all of our procedures, but not helping them. We had to find out why the blood flow to the rest of the body was so high that it deprived the kidney of adequate flow. Maybe that was where we needed to focus.

Blood flow to the liver

The place to start was the liver itself. But circulation to the liver is complicated. I wondered whether liver disease affected the blood supply to the liver, and in turn reduced the blood supply to the kidney. The liver receives blood flow from two sources—the hepatic artery, which directly nourishes the liver, and the portal vein, which collects blood from the intestine and spleen and delivers it to the liver, presumably to cleanse it of unwanted substances (Figure II-2).

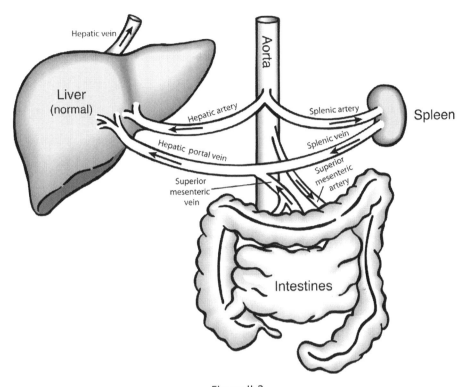

Figure II-2

The liver normally receives blood from both the hepatic artery and from the portal vein, which drains the intestines and spleen. Although the pressure is considerably higher in the hepatic artery than in the portal vein, most of the flow through a healthy liver is supplied by the portal vein.

When liver circulation is normal, blood in the portal vein—which is at a low pressure like most veins—flows easily through the liver capillaries that offer little resistance. In cirrhosis, however, scarring in the liver imposes a resistance to blood flow and the portal pressure rises (Figure II-3). This rising pressure leads to leakage of fluid out of the tributaries of the portal vein, and also encourages the opening of collateral blood vessels that seek an alternate route back to the heart without passing through the scarred liver. These collaterals, which often are in the esophagus (and called esophageal varices), may bleed in a life-threatening way.

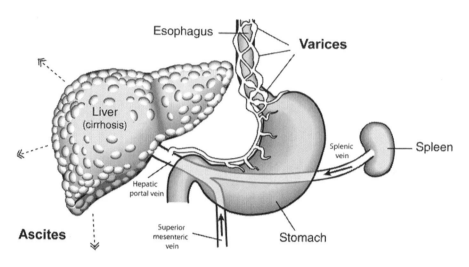

Figure II-3

Diagram of the liver circulation in cirrhosis. Elevated pressure in the liver and portal vein is thought to result from scarring in the liver, most commonly a complication of excess alcohol consumption. The high pressure causes "weeping" of fluid into the abdominal cavity (ascites) and opens fragile channels of blood seeking an alternative route back to the heart (varices).

But where does the high cardiac output come from in cirrhotics? Why is their cardiac output high while the kidneys are deprived of blood flow?

Some vascular bed must be at fault. The liver and portal circulation seemed to be the place to start.

If you want to measure blood flow through the liver by a technique similar to that we used in the kidney you can't use indocyanine green as the dye. This green dye is metabolized by the liver, so it would disappear before it leaves the liver. There would be no way to accurately calculate flow. Instead, we needed a substance that would stay in the blood stream so its concentration could be measured in the blood draining the liver.

Albumin stays in the circulation. I decided to use albumin labeled with an isotope of iodine that could be detected by a radiation detector. I set up a detector with a small well designed for sample tubes. By running plastic tubing through the well, it was possible to withdraw blood at a constant rate through the tubing and record the changing radioactivity in the blood as it passed through the well. When the albumin was injected and then withdrawn from the hepatic vein, a typical indicator dilution curve was recorded (Figure II-4). Knowing how much isotope we had injected, and knowing the concentration in the sampled blood over time, we could calculate the blood flow through the liver.

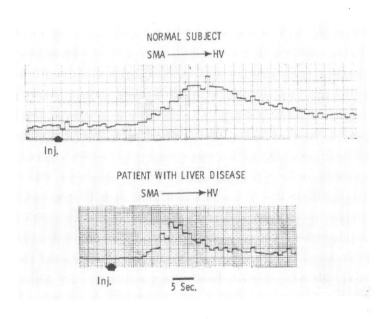

Figure II-4
Hepatic indicator-dilution curves recorded in blood withdrawn from the hepatic vein after injection of radioactive albumin into the superior mesenteric artery. Note that in the patient with liver disease the isotope appears far more quickly, thus indicating much higher flow through the liver in the presence of cirrhosis.

These ambitious, all-day hepatic studies were very demanding on the staff but remarkably well-tolerated by our cirrhotic patients who usually slept through them. The procedures provided remarkable new insights into the cirrhotic circulation. Since the radioactivity of the labeled albumin had a short half-life, the small doses we used had no long-term effects.

Working with two young Argentinian trainees, Roberto Groszmann and Bernardo Kotelanski, we found that the hepatic artery often delivered an extraordinarily high flow of blood to the liver, especially when the liver was inflamed by a recent alcohol binge. That was one source of high blood flow. Another was the mesenteric artery system that nourishes the intestine. High flow in this system often contributed to the high portal pressure that accounted for the abdominal swelling, and also supplied blood to alternate pathways that had opened, including the dreaded esophageal varices.

No one had previously shown that liver flow is increased in chronic liver disease. Why is this important? Efforts to deal with portal hypertension have primarily involved mechanical procedures to bypass the liver, assuming that obstruction to blood flow causes the dangerous elevation of portal pressure. But if high flow is contributing to the problem, efforts to reduce flow might be appropriate. In the 1970s, clinical studies were not exploring that possible therapeutic approach. Now, forty years later, interest has been rekindled because of evidence that nitric oxide, a gas released by the inner lining of arteries, may be the culprit in relaxing the arteries and causing excess blood flow in cirrhosis. We will deal more extensively with nitric oxide in later chapters.

Was the heart really innocent in progressive kidney failure? It appeared to be, since the cardiac filling pressure was low and the cardiac output high. And when we further increased output by increasing the blood volume, the kidney flow improved.

But we knew that alcohol excess can damage the heart muscle. Alcohol-induced heart failure was a common illness in our population. Could the heart be partly at fault, despite the high cardiac output? Did involvement of the liver somehow protect the heart from failing?

Since the blood pressure was low and the cardiac output high, the resistance in the circulation was low. In other words, the heart was working against a low resistance. (This will be discussed in greater detail in the next chapter.) What would happen if we raised resistance a little? Would the heart tolerate it, as a normal heart does? Or would it fail?

We infused angiotensin, a potent constrictor, in a series of patients with cirrhosis and apparently normal heart function. As the blood pressure rose only modestly to levels well within normal, the left ventricular filling pressure rose dramatically, often to as high as 30 mmHg. Yes, the heart was a major contributor to the hepatorenal syndrome. It limited the cardiac output and impaired kidney blood flow. In publishing our data I suggested that the name of the syndrome should be changed to "cardio-hepatorenal syndrome".

What is my specialty?

Because of my far-flung interest in the circulation to different organs, I had inadvertently developed three research teams, largely independent of each other except for my leadership role in all three. They were made up of young trainees who came from all over the world. The hypertension-kidney team included Manuel Velasquez from the Philippines, Sandy Logan from Canada and Ibrahim Khatri from Pakistan. They were interested in blood pressure and kidney function. The liver team consisted of Drs. Groszman and Kotelanski from Argentina as well as Nabil Guiha, who had left his Middle Eastern roots. They were preparing for academic careers. The heart team consisted of Constantinos Limas from Greece, Paul Hamosh from Israel, Ernesto Rodriguera from Brazil, Felix Tristani—who had migrated to the mainland from Puerto Rico—and Martin Broder, whose roots were in the States. They were dedicated to understanding heart function and were looking forward to cardiology careers. We had a remarkable "United Nations" and everyone worked well together.

At this time I was publishing papers in journals in three specialties and was invited to meetings all over the world in these three specialties. The downside of this popularity and influence was that my home life shrunk. Travel, along with night and weekend hours in the hospital, took me away from Syma and our three growing children. They all thrived but I felt increasingly guilty. My evenings at home were often occupied with analyzing reams of data collected during our studies. Having a spouse who nurtured the children and maintained home stability was a luxury. But there were frequent reminders of the failure of my father-ly responsibilities. My 8-year-old younger daughter confronted me one evening in my den, where I was working on a manuscript.

"Why do you have to work all the time?" she asked.

"Because I can't get all my work done during the day," I responded.

"Maybe you should ask them to put you in a slower group," she suggested helpfully.

My diverse activities were the problem. I had been following the blood flow to organs like the kidney and liver and finding that circula-tion abnormalities were key to many of the diseases that affected those organs. But medicine was becoming a profession of specialty silos. Clinical care was based on these silos. Gastroenterologists or liver spe-cialists didn't treat heart failure. Cardiologists were not interested in the liver. Kidney doctors were often dedicating their careers to dialysis for end-stage disease. My trainees were preparing for careers in their chosen specialties.

What was I? There was no specialty based on the circulation to vital organs. I could be a consultant to organ specialists when they suspected a blood flow problem, as I was at the V.A. Hospital. But this was not a recognized specialty and I would have no clinical colleagues.

An opportunity arose in 1974 to move to Minnesota and become a full-time cardiologist. This sounded attractive for the next stage of my career. Expansion of my program in Washington seemed unlikely. Funding for trainees, especially those who were non-citizens, was in-creasingly difficult to obtain. At a big Midwestern university, I thought, American trainees would flock to a creative research program and fund-ing would be more available.

I was aware of the downside of my move. I would take on far more administrative responsibilities, and I recognized that it may spell the end of my dabbling in nephrology and hepatology. The heart was too important an organ to short-change. It would require my undivided at-tention. I was ready to become a heart doctor.

CHAPTER III
Cardiac Function

My fascination with cardiac function and how it is affected by diseases and drugs made me want to pursue a career in cardiology. It was my group's innovative Washington studies on cardiac function that had identified me as a cardiologist to my academic colleagues and led to my recruitment to the University of Minnesota—not to become a cardiologist, but to assume the role of chief of cardiology. Since much of the work I would subsequently pursue in Minnesota was dependent on an understanding of the complexity of cardiac function, a brief review of this topic is in order.

In the 1960s, our understanding of how to control cardiac function was based on the standard medical school teaching that originated in studies of isolated hearts attributed to Otto Frank and Ernest Starling, who gathered the data for the cardiac function curve in Figure III-1.

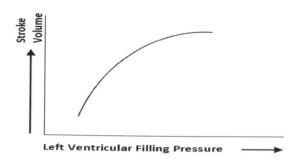

Figure III-1

Ventricular function is defined as the relationship between left ventricular filling pressure (or left ventricular stretch) and the subsequent force of contraction as defined by the volume of blood ejected (stroke volume). The curve relates increments in filling pressure to increments in stroke volume. The shape of this Starling Curve shows that at low filling pressures small increments of pressure or stretch produce large increases in force of contraction or stroke volume. As the filling pressure rises, however, the increment in stroke volume becomes less and eventually plateaus so that further increases in filling pressure do not result in a further increase in heart function.

The simple concept, which Frank and Starling and others had confirmed, was that the normal heart has the unique ability to pump harder when more blood is presented to it. That means that the heart can alter its force of contraction in response to changing demands. For example, if you stamp your feet while standing up, you deliver more blood to the heart from the lower extremities. This increased filling of the heart is immediately responded to by an increase in the force of contraction that delivers more blood on the next beat, an increase in what we call stroke volume.

What a deliciously efficient pumping system, never to be replicated by any mechanical device. It is a perfect pump. When more work is needed, it detects the increased demand and responds with more effort.

What is the biological process that accomplishes that adjustment? Exercise is the most common example. As we start to run, the muscles in the legs contract, mobilizing blood from the veins in the muscles and pumping it up to the heart. This is the so-called venous return. An increase in venous return acutely distends the heart, which senses this expansion and increases the force of the subsequent contraction.

No mechanical system could do that so precisely.

How does the heart detect that distention, and how does it adjust its contraction? Early studies in isolated heart muscle demonstrated that when the relaxed muscle is stretched with a weight, the subsequent contraction of the muscle is more forceful. That stretch in the relaxed state, which is similar to the interval between heart beats (diastole), is called preload. We now know that preload influences the length of sarcomeres, the microscopic building blocks of the myocardium, or heart muscle (Figure III-2).

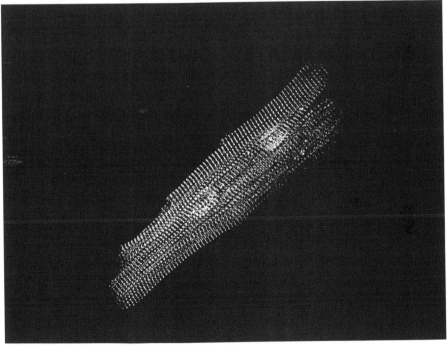

Figure III-2

A myocyte (heart muscle cell) from a dog is similar to that in man. This myocyte has two nuclei stained yellow (brighter spots). The sarcomeres, the contracting element of the cell, are lined up in a symmetrical arrangement. Since the space between sarcomeres is fixed, enlargement of the cell, which occurs in heart failure, is dependent on the synthesis of new sarcomeres.

This stretching of sarcomeres activates more calcium release. It is calcium that controls the force of contraction. It is a process about which we know much but still have more to learn.

The heart as a source of hormones

We now know that the heart is more than a pump. It also releases hormones, much like the adrenal or thyroid glands. These glands release hormones into the blood that circulate to all tissues of the body and affect their function. When the volume in the heart increases acutely because of an increase in blood returning from the veins to the heart, not only are the sarcomeres stretched but a variety of hormonal substances are released that may impact not only the heart itself but also the kidneys.

A hormone called natriuretic peptide ("natriuretic" means excreting more sodium in the urine) instructs the kidneys to begin eliminating any excess body fluid that might have been the cause of the increased cardiac filling. Some of these hormones also may stimulate a process of cardiac growth to deal with what could be a long-term demand for increased heart work. Therefore, a number of mechanisms influence the function and structure of the heart. But momentary changes in preload, as depicted in Figure III-1, are defined by the Frank-Starling curve. When preload increases, the force of contraction also increases. The converse is also true. When the heart is under-filled, as it was in Edward Cronin, the force of contraction is reduced and the patient may suffer from inadequate blood flow or shock.

Cardiac function only becomes an important issue when it is impaired. That means that the Frank-Starling curve has become depressed downward and to the right, as shown in Figure III-3. As noted in the figure, the output from the heart will be lower than normal for any given filling pressure.

It's critical to understand cardiac function when dealing with a sick patient: Does the patient need more volume to raise filling pressure, as was the case with Mr. Cronin, or does something need to be done to improve heart function? In Mr. Cronin's case, rapid volume expansion to raise the filling pressure restored cardiac output, so his cardiac function was normal. When an increase in filling pressure fails to restore cardiac output, the fault can be attributed to the heart and we can call it heart failure.

Under those circumstances we need to improve heart function by shifting the Frank-Starling curve upward and to the left (Figure III-3). That was likely the problem when Sam Farber experienced his severe heart failure. There was little we could do to improve cardiac function in 1957, even if we had been able to identify the problem.

What are the causes of depressed cardiac function? The most common cause in Western society is a deficiency in blood flow to nourish the heart muscle. Narrowing or obstruction of the coronary arteries is usually a consequence of atherosclerosis, the condition that led to Sam Farber's heart attack. Viral infections of the heart muscle also can cause depressed cardiac function. A chronically overworked heart as a result of high blood pressure, or an obstructed or leaky heart valve, can also be the culprit.

In the 1960s, the traditional view held that the only way to shift the Frank-Starling curve upward and to the left was to administer a so-called positive inotropic drug. Inotropism is the property that increases the force of contraction independent of preload (Figure III-3). You will also note in the figure the arrow marked V, or vasodilators, as another means of restoring cardiac function. That mechanism was not appreciated until 1972 and will be discussed more thoroughly later in this chapter.

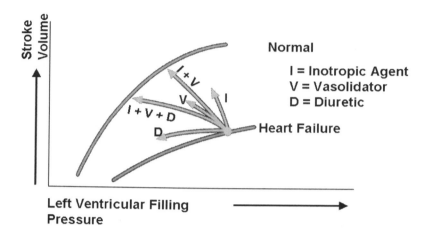

Figure III-3

The left ventricular function curve is shifted in heart failure downward and to the right from the normal curve shown in Figure III-1. Under those circumstances, even a rise in filling pressure will not increase stroke volume or cardiac output enough to provide nourishment to the body. Diuretics (D) will reduce blood volume and lower the elevated filling pressure. This may relieve the pressure build-up behind the heart and relieve congestive symptoms, but at the cost of a further fall in stroke volume. Shifting the curve upward and to the left is the therapeutic goal. Inotropic agents (I) are the traditional approach, but vasodilators (V), as described later in this chapter, can accomplish the same thing. All three classes of drugs can produce additive benefits by shifting the depressed curve upward and to the left.

The sympathetic nervous system exerts a potent stimulator effect on cardiac function (inotropism) and has been thought to be the prime natural mediator of inotropism. Noradrenaline or norepinephrine is the hormone released by the sympathetic nervous system when activated by stress or exercise. A synthetic version of this hormone has long been available as a drug called Levophed. That is the very drug that Sam Farber was given in a futile attempt to reverse his shock and that in Edward Cronin's case had almost killed him.

It is true that the Levophed increases the force of the heart's contraction, but its adverse effects on arteries and heart rhythm counteract any favorable effect on the Frank-Starling curve. What it does—and this is why it continues to be used—is raise blood pressure from dangerously low levels by constricting the arteries and increasing resistance. This rise in blood pressure may restore blood flow to the brain in a patient who has become drowsy or unconscious. It also makes care givers more comfortable.

Several laboratories were searching for drugs that could improve cardiac function without these other adverse effects. Some of these drugs became available for clinical research and we studied them after I moved to Minnesota hoping to identify one that could help patients suffering from inadequate blood flow that could not be restored with volume expansion. Although some of the drugs were successful in raising cardiac output and reversing the low output state in such patients, the infusion could not easily be continued over time, and side effects—including potentially lethal heart rhythm disturbances—frequently required stopping the infusion. We have not to this day found a potent and safe inotropic drug that can chronically improve depressed cardiac function.

I was committed to understanding the mechanism of the circulatory abnormality in sick patients in order to develop effective therapy, but there was a major problem to overcome. Some diseases predominantly affect the left ventricle and some predominantly the right ventricle. As shown in Figure III-4 the two ventricles are separated by the circulation to the lungs. Our early studies in the 1960s didn't really assess left ventricular function because we were measuring filling pressure of the right ventricle with a catheter passed into the right atrium. In order to measure filling pressure of the left ventricle to evaluate left ventricular function we would have to approach the left atrium, which was inaccessible from the veins.

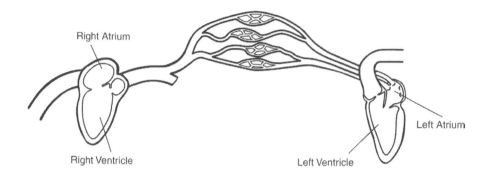

Figure III-4

The left ventricle is separated from the right ventricle by the lung. Obstruction of the lung circulation or damage to the right ventricle would impair the Starling curve of the right ventricle and provide no insight into that of the left ventricle. Furthermore, acute damage to the left ventricle may result in impaired left ventricular function that might not be detected by measuring right ventricular function.

The Frank-Starling curve for the right ventricle is independent from that of the left ventricle. If one ventricle is damaged or asked to perform excess work, measuring the filling pressure of the other ventricle could give misleading information. Fortunately, we had developed in 1969 a method for catheterization of the left ventricle at the bedside, a procedure described in Chapter 1. We now were in a position to go to the bedside and measure not only right heart filling pressure, but also left heart filling pressure. Thus we could independently assess the function of the right ventricle and the left ventricle and more precisely define the site of the abnormality.

After studying more than 30 patients with shock, it became apparent that shock with depressed cardiac function was not a single entity but was dependent on the cause. In patients with infections, either both ventricles were normal and responded favorably to volume expansion or both were abnormal because of the infection damaging the muscle. In these situations, the right ventricular filling pressure was not misleading. When it was low, so was the left ventricular filling pressure. When it was high, the left-sided pressure was high as well. When shock was due to an event in the lung circulation, such as massive clots (pulmonary embolism) obstructing the pulmonary arteries, then the problem was confined to the right ventricle, which was now failing, whereas the left ventricle was often under-filled and needing only more volume. When our studies identified this problem we could help the patient's cardiac output and blood pressure by expanding their blood even though the right heart filling pressure was elevated.

When shock was the consequence of an acute heart attack, or myocardial infarction, which almost always involves injury to the left ventricle, the problem could be isolated to the left ventricle. In those situations, the right ventricular filling pressure could be very misleading. The left heart had failed, but not the right. The right-sided pressure might not detect the acute problem in the left ventricle.

We were thus in a far better position to understand the nature of the circulatory problem in these patients who, up until the time we arrived on the scene, were being treated similarly and were often dying without being given a chance at effective therapy. We had made great strides in solving the diagnostic problem. But we really didn't know how to improve the function of the failing left ventricle. When a heart attack caused severe left ventricular failure, we had no drugs that could correct the problem. We could now pinpoint the problem to the left ventricle, but we couldn't do anything about it. Severe left ventricular failure after an acute MI was a death sentence.

A new insight

If fluid dynamic experts were to examine the Frank-Starling curve (Figure III-1), which defines left ventricular pump function, they would notice something missing. The factors influencing pump contraction are depicted (that is, preload or filling pressure and contractility or intrinsic muscle function), but there is no representation of the resistance or load against which the pump is emptying. Does this suggest that the pump function is independent of the load?

In isolated muscle studies the load can be set, usually by introducing a weight which the muscle must lift when it contracts. In an isolated heart study, the heart empties against a resistance—which can be varied—and will determine in part the pressure the heart generates. Does the function of the muscle decline when the weight is increased, and does the function of the heart decline when the resistance is raised?

Early studies were carried out in normal animal hearts. Under those circumstances, the heart seemed capable of adjusting the force of its contraction to meet the higher workload of a heightened load or resistance. Many of these elegant animal studies were performed at the National Institutes of Health in the laboratory of the late Stanley Sarnoff. Stan was a remarkably innovative and meticulous investigator who helped train many of the leading investigative cardiologists of the past generation. He noted the ability of these experimental hearts to miraculously adjust their contraction against varying loads and maintain a constant output. He thought it was an "autoregulatory" effect, meaning only that it was a mysterious mechanism by which the heart could maintain blood flow independent of the load. He even termed it "homeometric autoregulation", because he thought the heart accomplished this remarkable adjustment without altering its size, thus "homeometric".

If Sarnoff was right, the Frank-Starling curves did not need a representation for load. But Frank, Starling and Sarnoff were dealing with normal hearts. When we began studying patients with heart disease, a whole new physiology emerged.

High blood pressure puts a great demand on the left ventricle, which now must pump blood against a higher resistance or pressure when the ventricle begins to empty during systole. This burden causes the pumping chamber of the heart—the muscular wall of the left ventricle—to thicken or hypertrophy. Heart muscle fibers thicken, just as when the skeletal muscle-building exercise of weight lifting creates the sculpted bodies that are now so familiar at our gyms and beaches. The thicker heart muscle allows the heart to contract against the higher pressure of hypertension, just as the thicker skeletal muscle supports greater weight lifting.

The problem with heart hypertrophy is that it seems to be associated with complications. Although the hypertrophied muscle may be able to accomplish more work, and thus pump more effectively against the high pressure of hypertension, the thickened wall also requires more blood flow for nourishment. The coronary arteries, which are the sole source of blood flow to the heart muscle, cannot easily adapt to the increased flow demand. Furthermore, this increased muscle mass is a challenge to the electrical impulse that fires through the heart with each beat to instruct the heart to contract. When the muscle mass is increased, that electrical impulse must take a more circuitous route through the heart muscle and that may lead to electrical instability, heart rhythm disturbances, and even sudden death. So it has generally been assumed that hypertrophy of the heart, though a necessary accompaniment of long standing hypertension, is harmful. Interestingly, the hypertrophy that accompanies routine vigorous exercise apparently is not harmful, and is reversible when the exercise program is terminated.

The relationship between hypertension and heart failure has been known for a number of years through insurance statistics and epidemiologic studies in populations, but it was not clear that blood pressure itself was a contributor to heart failure. It was generally assumed that the hypertrophy of the heart muscle, the inadequacy of blood flow in the coronary arteries, and the superimposition of obstructing plaques in coronary arteries were major factors in the link between high blood pressure and heart failure. As noted previously, the Frank-Starling curve—which was the gold standard for the description of heart function—disregarded blood pressure or resistance to left ventricular emptying. Therefore, the assumption was that blood pressure itself did not influence heart function.

A revolutionary therapy

After our success in diagnosing unsuspected heart failure by catheterizing the left ventricle in Stanley Williams—our hypertensive patient described in Chapter 1—I was fascinated by the possibility that the pressure itself was contributing to this apparent heart failure. We set out to study the effect of acutely reducing blood pressure on the performance of the left ventricle. It seemed a simple undertaking, but I had to find the proper medication to safely lower blood pressure without affecting other determinants of heart function. What I needed was a drug that relaxed the arteries and would lower blood pressure, but which had no effect on sympathetic nervous impulses to the heart, nor any direct effect on the force of heart contraction.

In those days, most of the drugs that we were using to treat hypertension were thought to have direct cardiac effects, often by inhibiting sympathetic nervous system activity that would depress heart function, or by directly stimulating the heart. I recalled that there had been a report of the use of a chemical called sodium nitroprusside. This chemical could acutely lower severely elevated blood pressure that was threatening to damage the arteries nourishing the brain and heart. I obtained some of the chemical in powder form from a company that was making it for industrial purposes. To infuse it into patients, we had to sterilize it by passing it through a micropore filter to remove bacteria. It was, of course, not approved for clinical use, but in 1972 investigational use within your own institution required no special approval.

I also needed to prove that the drug could lower blood pressure without directly affecting the heart. To prove that hypothesis I turned to an experimental dog model. Dogs were widely used to address important research questions. The supplier of our experimental dogs obtained them from pounds just before they would have been euthanized. They provided valuable research information and often became pets of the laboratory personnel.

We anesthetized a dog and performed heart surgery, which involved threading a fine catheter into a branch of a coronary artery. The force of contraction of the heart muscle was assessed by a force transducer that we sutured onto the wall of the heart to monitor contraction with each beat. If one injects a drug into a coronary artery branch that nourishes a localized segment of the heart muscle, it is possible to assess the direct effects of the drug on the heart muscle independent of effects of the drug on the rest of the body. If the drug either stimulates or depresses the heart muscle directly, the force of contraction measured by the transducer will either increase or decrease. The question was this— if nitroprusside is injected into that coronary artery branch will there be an alteration in the muscle contraction?

We injected a series of doses of nitroprusside into the coronary artery. Muscle contraction was not altered. We concluded that nitroprusside had no direct effect on the heart muscle and that we could use it intravenously to lower blood pressure with confidence that the change in heart function observed would be a consequence of the blood pressure change, not a direct effect of the drug on the heart muscle.

We embarked on a study in a series of patients with severe hypertension who were admitted to the hospital for treatment of their blood pressure, but who had no obvious symptoms of heart failure. We identified eligible patients at the time of their admission so that we could rapidly perform the studies and then participate in their management. This required close cooperation of the medical staff in the V.A. Hospital who, fortunately, shared in our enthusiasm about improving management.

By the time we had studied 10 patients, we had our answer—and it was exciting. Five of the 10 patients had normal left ventricular function despite their high blood pressure. As we lowered their blood pressures, the function of their hearts remained unchanged. In fact, nitroprusside also lowered their heart filling pressures by decreasing venous return. Their cardiac output dropped as their filling pressure fell, just as predicted by the Frank Starling curve (Fig III-1).

Sarnoff was right. Pressure is not a determinant of heart function when the heart is functioning normally, as it was in his animal models. However, in the five hypertensive patients who had abnormal left ventricular function similar to Stanley Williams' condition, reduction of blood pressure with nitroprusside produced a marked improvement in their depressed heart function. Thus, the failing heart—in contrast to the normal heart, is very sensitive to pressure. In these patients, pressure itself appeared to be a major contributor to heart failure.

There was one additional observation that would lead to a profound change in the way we think about pressure and heart function. While infusing nitroprusside in these five patients with heart failure, we found that the improvement in heart function could be demonstrated long before the blood pressure began to fall. That is, infusing the drug was associated with a progressive improvement in heart function even before the dose had been increased to a level that reduced blood pressure. We were also monitoring the arterial waveform from a needle placed in an artery in these patients. The shape of the waveform changed dramatically long before the blood pressure began to fall. This was, in fact, the observation that led us to develop the method for waveform analysis that eventually resulted in the CV Profilor instrument described in Chapter 1.

Therefore, it wasn't just the blood pressure that was the culprit, but something more profound. Indeed, the blood pressure is in part determined by the heart's contraction, so the pressure can't be viewed as simply an opposition to the ventricle's delivery of a stroke volume. That total opposition to emptying of the left ventricle has to be captured in a term like "impedance", which is adopted from electrical circuitry and refers to the total forces opposing the emptying of the left ventricle with each beat. Clearly, nitroprusside was reducing that impedance before it reduced the pressure itself. That meant that the ventricle was increasing its output and maintaining pressure while the impedance and resistant was falling in response to the drug.

An impedance curve, as shown in Figure III-5, now needed to supplement the Frank-Starling curve in depiction of cardiac function. This previously unrecognized role for impedance is what accounts for the arrow pointing upward and to the left on the Starling curve and labeled V for vasodilator in Figure III-3.

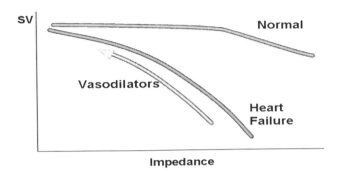

Figure III-5

Although an increase of impedance does not affect stroke volume in the normal heart until it reaches high levels that do not ordinarily occur, the failing heart is exquisitely sensitive to even modest increases in impedance. Vasodilators that reduce imped- ance can profoundly improve function of the failing heart.

How does impedance differ from blood pressure?

Blood pressure is the product of cardiac output and systemic vascu- lar resistance (BP=(CO) X (SVR). If the output goes up and the resis- tance stays the same, the blood pressure will rise. If the resistance falls in response to a drug and the output simultaneously rises, then the blood pressure may stay the same even though the resistance has fallen and the impedance to left ventricular ejection has now been reduced. Thus the secret of the relationship between the blood vessels and the heart was not necessarily the role of pressure but the role of the sum of the forces opposing left ventricular emptying which I called impedance.

Could an impedance load have accounted for Sam Farber's termi- nal heart failure and shock, which we were unable to reverse? If I had understood in 1956 what I had learned 16 years later, and if I had had a source of nitroprusside at that earlier time, perhaps Sam would have survived. The thought haunted me.

To say that I was preoccupied by these exciting ideas would be an understatement. I couldn't really share them with my family. Syma was in graduate school in art history at the University of Maryland. The physiology of cardiac function was not of interest to her. I may have made some feeble attempts at explaining what I had learned, but our conversations were always interrupted by the pressing needs of family life. Our three children were entering their teens with diverse interests and activities. I really couldn't share any of my excitement with them because the concepts required too much background in physiology and clinical medicine. I tried to pay attention to everyone's interests and activities, but my thoughts were often elsewhere.

As I thought more deeply about our concept that the function of the heart could be profoundly influenced by the load against which it is pumping, I came to the growing realization that this whole new therapeutic approach needed to be thoroughly tested. Whether it was to be called "impedance reduction therapy" or "vasodilator therapy", I believed it could revolutionize the management of the failing heart. What I could not know in 1972 was that I would not undertake the study of this new concept at the VA Hospital in Washington, but at the University of Minnesota in Minneapolis.

CHAPTER IV
Acute Myocardial Infarction

I was first introduced to acute myocardial infarction in 1949 during my freshman year at Union College. My mother developed severe chest pain and her doctor, a fine internist who had become a family friend, rushed to the house and announced that she had suffered a "coronary thrombosis". The ambulance came to take her to the hospital where she remained for six weeks.

That simple timeline does nothing to describe the family turmoil surrounding this event. When we were not in the hospital visiting mother, our house became a mausoleum dedicated to her memory. Mom had never been away. The house and all of its activities had been under her control. We tread quietly. There was no radio and no laughter. Meals, which my father, who was City Manager of Schenectady, N.Y., my older sister Grace and I all helped to prepare, were somber affairs. Our cocker spaniel, whose dedication to my mother included growling at me if I raised my voice to her, spent most of his day perched at the end of the sidewalk where the ambulance had taken her away. Mom's condition was viewed as grave.

Uncle Harry (Harry Gold) was summoned from New York and made a grand entrance to Ellis Hospital. The staff had been forewarned that the great cardiologist from New York was coming. He lived up to his advance billing, examining the chart with great flourish, reviewing the electrocardiograms, visiting his sister at the bedside, and then sagely announcing that she should be treated with warfarin.

Blood clots and heart attacks

Warfarin, or coumadin, is an anticoagulant; that is, it prevents blood from clotting. It was also used as a rat poison because it causes rats to hemorrhage internally and fatally. The very name "coronary thrombosis" implies that a clot in the coronary artery had caused the event, which was damage to the heart muscle in the area nourished by that coronary artery. It seemed only logical that a drug to prevent clotting would be an appropriate choice. Furthermore, a clinical trial published in 1948—one of the first large trials in cardiology—had demonstrated the beneficial effects of warfarin in patients with coronary thrombosis. That trial had been organized by a friend of Harry's, Dr. Irving Wright, who was an elegant and somewhat arrogant Cornell University senior physician. I subsequently got to know him when I was a medical student at Cornell.

Wright had overseen a trial supported by the American Heart Association that studied more than 1000 patients with coronary thrombosis. The patients were randomly assigned to receive either warfarin or a placebo. The therapy was blinded so that neither the patient nor the medical staff knew which treatment the patient had been given. When the data were analyzed, it was found that 23.4 per cent of the control group who received placebo had died, but only 16 per cent of the warfarin-treated patients had died. No one expected the drug to prevent all deaths, but this reduction in mortality was the equivalent of saving almost 80 lives for every 1000 patients treated. Although there were some bleeding complications in the warfarin group, the benefit appeared substantial. Harry's recommendation was therefore well-supported by evidence.

There was a problem, however, with administering warfarin. The drug's effect and dosage adjustment had to be monitored by a blood at least twice a week. Harry did not trust the lab in this local hospital, an attitude that was not well received by the hospital staff. This was a particularly sensitive issue because the laboratory director was a family friend. Nonetheless, Harry made arrangements for my mother's prothrombin time test to be performed at the Albany Medical Center, which was part of Albany Medical School.

On the mornings of the scheduled tests, I drove to Ellis Hospital, picked up the blood sample, transported it the 15 miles to Albany, delivered it to the laboratory, waited for the result, and returned the result to Ellis Hospital where Dr. Horwitz would prescribe the day's dose of warfarin.

The saga of warfarin's role in the management of this disease has had its ups and downs. Wright's trial was subsequently discounted when it was learned that the participating staffs could look at the packets of so-called "blinded" medications and identify which was warfarin and which was placebo. Since the packets were prescribed sequentially, it was possible to know before randomization whether the patient was going to receive warfarin or placebo. The medical team could therefore decide not to enter a patient if he or she were destined to receive the treatment they did not favor. Or a staff member could wait to enter a patient until the next packet was the desired treatment. No one could really be certain how this "unblinding" could have influenced the results, but the study's credibility was lost.

All future controlled trials were designed to randomize therapy numerically; that is, a number is assigned to a patient who matched the number on a medication packet. The number is not assigned until the patient is randomized. Therefore the staff cannot identify the medication packet until the patient has already been entered into the study.

But that wasn't the only problem with the attractive hypothesis that anticoagulants are good for heart attacks. Pathologists began examining the hearts of patients who died in the acute phase of their "coronary thrombosis" and often found no clots in the coronary arteries. A belief was evolving that clots do not cause heart attacks. The diagnosis "coronary thrombosis" was forever changed to "acute myocardial infarction" or "AMI", implying that the problem was damage to heart muscle, but that the mechanism of the damage was not necessarily known. It was not until years later, with the advent of arteriography to visualize the lumen of the coronary arteries with dye, that the truth became known.

Marcus DeWood, an aggressive young cardiologist from Seattle, was the first to carry out angiography in patients while they were suffering from an AMI. He demonstrated in 1980 that most acute myocardial infarctions are indeed caused by clots superimposed on underlying cholesterol-containing plaques in the coronary arteries. The plaques may have existed for years and be quite small, causing no symptoms. The clot, however, is new. Pathologists often missed the clots because they tend to dissolve by themselves over time after the damage has been done.

What about anticoagulants? Aren't they now restored to their rightful place in management of AMI? Not really. Warfarin doesn't dissolve clots. It only prevents new clots. Clots that previously existed had already caused damage.

New drugs that dissolve existing clots became available in more recent years and are now standard therapy for AMI. These are thrombolytics, not anticoagulants. Furthermore, warfarin appears not even to be very effective in preventing clots in coronary arteries. Newer drugs—even aspirin—more directly affect the clotting mechanism in arteries and have become treatments of choice to prevent coronary thrombosis.

Then why did warfarin appear to benefit patients with AMI in the earlier study? It probably had much to do with the way we treated MI in the past. My mother's 6-week hospitalization at bed rest was standard therapy. Lying in bed for six weeks encourages clots to form—not in the arteries, but in the veins that drain the legs. These clots in the lower extremities may break off and travel to the heart and lungs where they can cause serious mischief, including death. The standard treatment then and now for venous clots or thrombophlebitis is warfarin, because the mechanism of venous clot formation is different from that in arteries.

Wright may have been right. But we no longer keep patients in bed after an AMI. Early ambulation prevents the clots in the legs. No routine warfarin. At least not in the first part of the 21st century.

My mother made a rather uneventful recovery, either because of, or in spite of, my shuttle service to Albany. Her return to the house was a major family event. Bruce became his old canine self, but now even growled louder if he felt Mom was threatened. My father became more solicitous of her every need. We tried not to trouble her. She remained a caring and thoughtful counselor for everyone in her extended family who sought her help. She died 15 years later of a stroke, long after the family home had been sold, the dog had died, and my sister and I had dispersed. My father could never quite adjust to her loss.

The complications of myocardial infarction

Not knowing what caused MI's was not the only deficiency in our knowledge about this catastrophic disease when I started my internship in 1956. As with Sam Farber, we didn't know how to treat it, we didn't understand the complications, and we were woefully incapable of altering the outcome. Passivity was the standard approach, and acceptance of the inevitable was a substitute for inquisitiveness.

I never forgot the experience with Sam, whose disease silently worsened to the point of severe heart failure after he left the hospital after what appeared to be an uncomplicated AMI. Over the next few years I observed several other patients who had been discharged after a heart attack only to return months or years later with enlargement of their heart and symptoms of heart failure that carried with it a bleak prognosis. Others, however, seemed to suffer no long-term effects of their previous heart attack. Angiography to visualize the coronary arteries and echocardiography to image the heart chambers eventually came into use, but even these technological advances could not explain why the disease progressed in some but not others. Little if anything of pertinence appeared in the literature.

As I traversed the medical wards of the V.A. Hospital in the late 1960s, now armed with my cart to perform bedside hemodynamic studies, I couldn't resist the idea of finding out what actually was happening to a patient with an AMI. Could it be that we were missing something important with our crude clinical evaluations? Was there something measurable in the acute phase of their illness that might give us insight into this later deterioration in some but not all patients?

To study the function of the left ventricle, we would need to catheterize the heart. But heart catheterization on a patient with AMI was a very sensitive and contentious issue. Patients admitted with AMI were put to bed and not molested. The goal was to keep them mildly sedated, pain free and quiet. The mere thought of putting tubes into their heart and agitating them with needles, instruments and noise was anathema to standard practice. How things have changed. Today, patients are whisked to the catheterization laboratory as soon as they arrive in the emergency room. Aggressive diagnostic and therapeutic efforts in patients with AMI are one of the primary activities of the cardiologist's day.

But in 1969 the world of cardiology was different. To bring my equipment to the bedside of a patient with an AMI would require a major educational effort and careful reassurance of both the patient and the health care workers. Was that reassurance justified? How did I know that the procedure could be safely accomplished?

Patient and institutional consent were needed to undertake the studies I proposed. Consent was relatively simple in those days. There was no Institutional Review Board, the professional and lay body that today serves to protect patients from experiments they may not understand. There was no formal informed consent process. There was only a brief explanation to the patient and his or her signed agreement to the procedure. More importantly, there was a compassionate physician intent on learning and confident that the procedure could be performed safely and that the new knowledge was worth the risk—even if the patient couldn't share fully in the decision.

Even then, however, I recognized that this potentially dangerous catheterization procedure needed knowledgeable peer review before it could be launched. A number of distinguished cardiologists around the country were queried by my institution. Most said it was potentially dangerous and unprecedented to put catheters in the hearts of patients in the acute stage of a heart attack. They would not themselves choose to do the procedure, but they agreed that the information to be obtained could be very useful. Most expressed support for *my* doing it! When my first report from these experiments was accepted for presentation at the prestigious annual clinical investigation meetings, then on the Boardwalk in Atlantic City, the president of the organization called me to be certain that we had performed these studies with institutional and professional approval.

The first experiences were revealing. Patients with acute MI suffered from left heart failure, even if they did not manifest heart failure symptoms. Filling pressures in the left ventricle were strikingly elevated, a finding that was not expected because of the absence of symptoms of heart failure. The patients were functioning on a depressed Frank-Starling curve (Figure III-3), but were not suffering from clinical signs of heart failure. There was no way on clinical examination or X-ray to detect that their left ventricle was dysfunctional.

When left is right

Actually, strikingly elevated left ventricular filling pressure was not always present in acute MI. We learned that the hard way. Henry Sampson, a 72-year-old man, was admitted with what appeared to be an acute myocardial infarction. His blood pressure was very low and he had what was thought to be early signs of shock. When we catheterized his heart we found that his left ventricular filling pressure was almost normal but his right heart filling pressure was high. This was not the pattern we had been seeing in acute MI. In fact the pattern was typical of a clot in the pulmonary artery (pulmonary embolism), which puts a burden on the right ventricle and often masquerades as acute MI. His electrocardiogram was consistent with pulmonary embolism. Since the management of pulmonary embolism is dramatically different than that of acute MI, we felt he needed emergency angiography by injecting dye into his pulmonary artery to identify the clot that could potentially be removed surgically.

There was no clot. His lung circulation looked normal. We didn't know what was causing his illness, and we had no idea how to treat it. His circulation gradually deteriorated and the poor man died.

I went to the autopsy room to examine the heart. The left ventricle looked quite normal, but the thin-walled right ventricle exhibited extensive damage. The right coronary artery, which nourishes the right ventricle, was occluded at its origin. The patient had suffered a right ventricular (RV) infarction.

RV infarctions had previously been reported as a rare autopsy finding but had never been diagnosed clinically. The frequency of the autopsy finding could not be determined because pathologists, when dissecting the heart, usually cut off and discarded the right ventricle without examining it. In their opinion, it was not the site of important disease.

We were ready to deal more effectively if we saw the same condition again. Jack Harwood was a 48-year-old V.A. administrator with a high-level job in the central office. He was transferred to our facility from another hospital 18 hours after admission with an apparent acute MI. His heart rate was slow on admission, his blood pressure was low at 90 mmHg and his neck veins were bulging, thus implying right ventricular failure. He was free of pain and not short of breath, but very weak. His electrocardiogram suggested a myocardial infarction in the back wall of the heart where the right ventricle resides. Everything pointed to a right ventricle (RV) infarction. Left heart pressures were normal, as predicted. It was clear to me that his left ventricle needed more volume in order to pump enough blood to support his blood pressure We aggressively infused fluids to increase his left ventricle (LV) filling pressure, even though his bulging neck veins would ordinarily indicate no more fluids. His blood pressure rose, his heart rhythm normalized and he made an uncomplicated recovery.

Could Jack Harwood have ended on the autopsy table, as did Henry Sampson? We'll never know, but Jack stopped by to see me regularly over the following years to express his appreciation in being the first known survivor of an RV infarction.

Over the next year we identified six other patients with RV filling pressures that exceeded LV filling pressures, now a hallmark of RV infarction. We knew what to do. Their left ventricles were under-filled because of the inability of the right ventricle to pump adequate blood. We needed to expand their blood volume to enhance filling of the left ventricle. None of them died.

In 1974, we reported our new clinical syndrome, right ventricular infarction, and also reported dog experiments we carried out to replicate the syndrome. For years afterward, whenever I went to an institution as a visiting professor, I would be presented a case of RV infarction, often referred to as "Cohn's Syndrome". I was credited with saving a lot of lives.

But what about the more common variety of acute MI? What happened over time to those patients with a failing left ventricle ?

Recovery from a heart attack

I decided to address the question in 1971 with Martin Broder, a senior research fellow at the V.A. Hospital. We re-catheterized a group of patients a few weeks after they had recovered from the acute phase of their illness. We found that in some the LV filling pressure had returned to normal, but in others the pressure was still elevated even though they had no symptoms. Sam Farber was probably in the latter group of patients with a persistent functional deficit of the heart but without symptoms that we could detect before he went home. I still couldn't understand, though, why Sam had deteriorated over a six month period. Even if he had had unrecognized heart failure, why did it get progressively worse without any signs of further myocardial damage such as a new heart attack?

There was a potential physiologic basis for why reduced function of the left ventricle might induce further impairment in function over time. This mechanism occurred to me in 1970 when I collected the data from our studies. But it will require a pretty strong dose of physiology to explain it. Those not interested in mechanisms may skip the next four paragraphs and take my word that heart failure can beget more heart failure. But I hope most readers will want to understand it.

The wall of the left ventricle of the heart is about 1 cm (less than half an inch) thick. Most of this is muscle or myocardium. The myocardium, of course, is nourished by the coronary arteries that provide the energy for tissue health and muscle contraction. The arteries travel on the outer side of the myocardium, and their branches penetrate through the wall to the inner side of the muscle to provide nourishment to the whole wall (Figure IV-1).

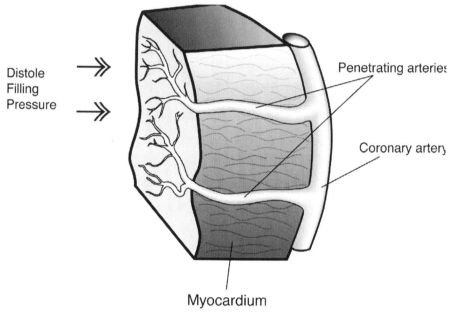

Distole
Filling
Pressure

Penetrating arteries

Coronary artery

Myocardium

Figure IV-1

Diagrammatical representation of blood flow to the heart muscle (myocardium). The coronary arteries travel on the outer surface of the heart, but nourishing the wall, which is about one cm. thick, and especially the inner portion of the wall requires flow through the penetrating arteries and into the capillaries bed that serves the inner wall or endocardium. Since the penetrating arteries are compressed by muscle contraction during systole, flow must occur during diastole, when the muscle is relaxed. During that period the capillaries in the inner layer or endocardium may be compressed by an elevated pressure inside the chamber, the ventricular diastolic pressure or filling pressure.

The problem with this design is that blood cannot penetrate through the wall when the muscle is contracting because the squeezing closes the small penetrating arteries. Therefore, all the nourishment of the working heart muscle must be delivered in diastole—during the interval when the heart is not contracting. Furthermore, the heart consumes a lot of energy with its rhythmic muscle contraction. The balance between oxygen delivery to the heart muscle and its oxygen consumption is very fragile. Indeed, because of the tenuous flow of blood in the penetrating arteries, the heart muscle extracts almost all the oxygen out of the blood nourishing it. It is quite distinct from other organs. When blood is collected from the veins draining other organs, the blood is only slightly darker than arterial blood, indicating that some of the oxygen has been removed in passing through the organ. When blood is collected from the coronary sinus—the blood vessel that drains the blood nourishing the heart—the blood is pitch black because the muscle has extracted almost all the oxygen. If blood flow is reduced, the heart cannot respond like other organs by extracting more oxygen because all the oxygen is gone. The result is that the heart is on the verge of ischemia—an inadequacy of blood flow—even when the circulation is normal.

Some years ago, a group of investigators performed electrocardiograms on apparently healthy young firemen immediately after they had run up and down ladders to put out fires. Their electrocardiograms revealed evidence of transient ischemia suggesting that the stress and heavy workload had demanded more blood flow than their healthy coronary arteries could deliver. The firemen, of course, recovered quickly during rest.

The inner layer of the heart muscle (the endocardium) is most in jeopardy from being inadequately nourished because the penetrating arteries must traverse the whole wall before getting blood to the endocardium. But there is a further impediment to endocardial blood flow. Pressure in the chamber of the heart that is directly in contact with the endocardium may further compress the penetrating arteries nourishing the muscle. When the pressure in the ventricle in diastole (the filling pressure) is normal, say five mmHg, it exerts no meaningful compressive force on the inner layer arteries. But when the filling pressure is elevated, as it was in our patients with AMI, it could further impair nourishment of the inner layer of the heart. That could lead to further impairment of heart function. I thought, perhaps that elevated filling pressure, especially if it was sustained, could have led to progressive heart failure and the deterioration that Sam experienced.

A test for revolutionary therapy

What could we do to safely lower that pressure in the left ventricle during diastole? I had recently completed our observations in hypertensive heart failure with the dramatic response to sodium nitroprusside, and recognized that nitroprusside appeared to improve left ventricular function even before the blood pressure had fallen. Based on this, I was enticed by the possibility that nitroprusside could become an effective means of treating the unrecognized heart failure of acute myocardial infarction.

Here we had another challenge to conventional thinking. These patients with acute myocardial infarction were not hypertensive. In fact, in this setting the main fear was that blood pressure might fall too low and the patient might develop shock. The idea of using a drug that lowers blood pressure was counterintuitive and not advised.

I will never forget our first experience. Morris Jackson was a 57-year-old overweight man with known diabetes. I first met him 12 hours after his admission following a call from his attending physician who knew of our research efforts. Morris was sweating profusely and propped up in bed to ease his breathing. He had been given morphine in an attempt to relieve his pain and was drowsy but still clutching his chest. He described the pressure sensation that went down both arms. His electrocardiogram showed the classical signs of an acute myocardial infarction involving the anterior wall of his left ventricle. The nurses were frequently recording his blood pressure using a cuff, and had recorded it at 106/70 mmHg—apparently much lower than his usual pressure, which his wife told us was about 150.

After discussing with his wife our planned approach and getting both her and the patient's approval we embarked on our hemodynamic studies. The left ventricular catheter revealed a filling pressure of 35 mmHg, three times normal. His cardiac output recorded by our indicator dilution technique was approximately three liters per minute, half what it should have been for a man of his size. Morris was in severe heart failure. When we placed a needle in his artery we recorded a blood pressure of 136/94, well within the upper normal range, even though the cuff reading taken by the nurse was considerably lower.

I felt we had an ideal patient to test our hypothesis that sodium nitroprusside would improve the function of his left ventricle. We started an infusion at our usual low initial dose. The LV filling pressure began to fall. As we gradually increased the dose of nitroprusside, the filling pressure in the heart fell further. In contrast, the pressure in the artery dropped only slightly to 124/76 mmHg.

We repeated the measurement of his cardiac output. It had gone up. We increased the rate of the infusion and the LV filling pressure fell to nearly normal. A repeat cardiac output measurement showed that the output had doubled from three to six liters per minute. We had dramatically lowered his impedance without significant lowering of blood pressure (Figure III-5).

His profuse sweating stopped. he became wide awake and claimed his breathing was much better and his pain had disappeared. His urine output, which had been scanty began to increase robustly. This meant that we had increased the blood flow to his kidneys. We had, in fact, successfully treated Morris' heart failure by using a vasodilator drug that improved the function of the acutely infarcted left ventricle without dangerously reducing blood pressure. The pain relief suggested that we had restored a balance between his heart muscle's consumption and delivery of oxygen. Yes, we may have reduced the work of the heart by relaxing his arteries, which in turn reduced impedance to emptying. But we also may have restored blood flow to the inner layers of the heart by reducing the compressive force of a high left ventricular filling pressure.

Over the following months we obtained similar results in other patients with AMI. I was anxious to get these remarkable observations published as soon as possible, because I had divulged the preliminary results of our studies at the November meeting of the American Heart Association, but in a session with no published abstract. Therefore, I had no priority on this observation until the data were published. We quickly prepared a manuscript describing the results in 20 patients studied, suggesting that this could be a new and important management strategy for patients with heart failure complicating AMI.

The highest profile journal was, and still is, *The New England Journal of Medicine*. I submitted the paper. Weeks went by without a response. I became concerned that this delay would jeopardize our priority on the concept. Finally, a letter from the Journal's editor, Franz Ingelfinger, arrived.

He had rejected the paper based on intense discussion at the Editorial Board meeting, he said. As a gastroenterologist, Dr. Ingelfinger had no particular expertise in the area of our research. He made that point in his letter (Figure IV-2) and revealed that although some members of the Editorial Board felt the study was provocative and should be published, the majority felt the concept and procedure was so dangerous that *The New England Journal of Medicine* should not publish it. He suggested, with remarkable clairvoyance, that perhaps the idea was so innovative that the traditionalists on his Editorial Board could not understand its importance.

The New England Journal of Medicine

10 SHATTUCK STREET, BOSTON, MASSACHUSETTS 02115—TELEPHONE 617 / 734-9800

OFFICIAL PUBLICATION OF THE MASSACHUSETTS MEDICAL SOCIETY

OFFICE OF THE EDITOR

January 12, 1972

#71-2176

Jay N. Cohn, M.D.
Veterans Administration Hospital
50 Irving Street, N.W.
Washington, D.C. 20422

Dear Dr. Cohn:

The Editorial Board of the Journal, I regret to say, did not recommend acceptance of the manuscript "Improved Left Ventricular Function During Nitroprusside Infusion in Acute Myocardial Infarction."

The paper was extensively discussed at the Board meeting, and I fear that the overwhelming opinion was not only that we should not publish it but that the procedure advocated might prvbe extremely dangerous, particularly in semi-skilled hands.

Of the expert reviewers who read the paper, one was quite negative and suggested that the hemodynamic effects of peripheral vasodilitation, particularly with respect to coronary circulation, have been studied by Gorlin and others. The other felt that the article was interesting and did present some original observations. He also, however, feared that "the potential hazards" of the procedure were such that we could not publish the paper unless it were accompanied by a strongly cautionary editorial.

As you know, I have no competence in the area of your paper, but it seems to me that either of two things must be true. Either your treatment is so novel and radical that the "establishment" members of our Board could not appreciate it; or, it is indeed a dangerous procedure that, many discussants felt, could lead to increase in the size of the infarcted area.

Sincerely yours,

Franz J. Ingelfinger, M.D.

FJI:kk
Enclosures

Figure IV-2

Rejection letter received from The New England Journal of Medicine. The typo in the second paragraph reminds us that it was a time before computer-based spell checking.

I was deflated but not discouraged. I knew we had an important new observation that would influence the future of cardiovascular medicine. I immediately sent the manuscript, without modification, to *Lancet*, the British journal which is comparable in prestige to *The New England Journal of Medicine* and the leading medical journal in the United Kingdom. *Lancet* accepted the manuscript for publication by return mail and published it soon thereafter.

The concept was now established in the literature. Left ventricular function was almost invariably impaired in AMI, and that dysfunction could be dramatically improved by infusion of sodium nitroprusside. But would the treatment save lives? Since there are about one million AMI's in the United States each year, a new treatment could have profound effects on health care.

We needed to find out if the treatment could have long-term beneficial effects. The method to accomplish such a study would be a clinical trial, the same approach that my mentor, Ed Freis, had used to establish the benefit of antihypertensive drug therapy in patients with hypertension.

My career as a clinical trialist was about to begin. At the same time, I was about to leave Washington for my new life in Minnesota.

CHAPTER V
The Study Without a Name

After publication of the favorable effects of nitroprusside on left ventricular function in patients with acute myocardial infarction, it was clear that we had to go the next step. We had shown that nitroprusside reduced an elevated left ventricular filling pressure and increased the cardiac output. This improvement in left ventricular function certainly corrected the abnormal state we had identified in our patients with acute myocardial infarction. It also appeared to improve patients' immediate well-being by relieving shortness of breath, often relieving chest pain and improving kidney function as well. Signs of impaired blood flow, such as sweating and confusion, were also relieved.

But many of our patients had no obvious symptoms of impaired heart function. Did these patients also benefit from the nitroprusside infusion? By normalizing the elevated left ventricular filling pressure, did we improve blood flow to the inner layers of the heart muscle? If so, would this lead to long-term benefit by preventing further heart muscle damage? Had nitroprusside been infused in Sam Farber at the time of his acute MI could his subsequent heart failure have been prevented?

A clinical trial plan

We not only had to show that the heart was functioning better, but that the outcome was improved. This would be a far more formidable venture. We needed a large population of patients in whom we could intervene with the drug or placebo and demonstrate that patients who received the drug benefited in terms of mortality or long-term morbidity. This was certainly not a study that we could undertake in a single center.

Fortunately I had the experience of watching my mentor, Ed Freis, carry out a multicenter study in hypertensive patients to demonstrate that a drug therapy which lowers blood pressure has a beneficial effect on outcome. This was the model I needed to undertake the definitive study. Ed had used the V.A. Cooperative Studies program to fund his trial. In 1973 I was still a full-time V.A. physician in Washington, so I turned to that same source.

The Cooperative Studies program was an innovative research endeavor still in its infancy. The program's goal was to identify problems that affected veterans' health that could potentially be enhanced by new therapies that needed testing. This program allowed investigators from a number of V.A. medical centers to band together, develop a common protocol, and undertake trials with V.A. support. It was an ideal mechanism to support our proposal, since myocardial infarction was a lethal condition in V.A. hospitals and there was no treatment being administered for it.

The concept that clots in the coronary artery caused the infarction had yet to emerge, so techniques and tools for dissolving or obliterating the clots had yet to be developed. Drugs that we now know can alter the course of the disease had not been studied. In the early 1970s, time was the only treatment. We were proposing an aggressive management strategy that we thought might be effective in minimizing heart damage and improving outcomes. It was a bold approach to a common and serious disease that had not previously been subjected to such invasive management.

I submitted a draft of a preliminary protocol. The Cooperative Studies evaluation committee agreed to support a planning process that allowed me to bring together several potential investigators and a biostatistician from the V.A. The beauty of this Cooperative Studies program was that the V.A. provided not only support for carrying out the work, but also provided a biostatistical support center that could collect and analyze the data.

In our initial meetings we reached several important conclusions. Since our therapy was designed to improve left ventricular function, it was imperative that the trial include only patients who had evidence of fairly severe left ventricular failure. This meant that we had to document the presence of left ventricular failure in all patients entered into the trial. And, as we had already shown, heart failure could not be identified by signs and symptoms. We would need to document heart failure with a catheter in the heart. Furthermore, since the infusion rate of nitroprusside had to be individualized in order to improve heart function, we needed to monitor the LV filling pressure during the infusion to optimize management and document the improvement in function.

We had been using our bedside left ventricular catheterization technique to study patients, but this was a procedure used only by us. I felt the technique would be unsuitable for application in other hospitals with less experienced investigators. We needed a more practical way to monitor left ventricular function.

Monitoring the heart's filling pressure

In 1970, a group of investigators from Los Angeles, led by a friend named Willie Ganz, had developed a catheter that could be inserted into a vein and be carried by the flowing blood through the heart into the pulmonary artery that leads from the right ventricle toward the left ventricle. It had long been known that a catheter advanced into a small branch of a pulmonary artery could be wedged deep into the artery and provide a pressure equal to that in the left atrium (Figure V-1). The reason for this is that when the catheter is plugged into a small pulmonary artery, the blood flow is blocked and the column of blood between the tip of the catheter and the left atrium becomes stagnant. Since the left atrium has a pressure equal to the filling pressure of the left ventricle, this pulmonary wedge pressure becomes a measure of left ventricular filling pressure. For many years when the left ventricle was inaccessible in heart catheterizations, the pulmonary wedge pressure was recorded to provide a guide to the function of the left ventricle.

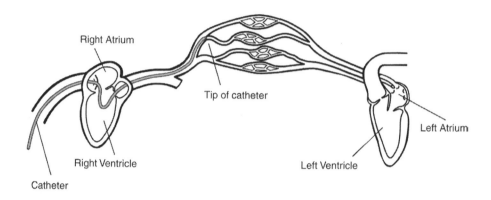

Figure V-1

Diagrammatical representation of the position of a catheter passed from a vein through the right atrium and right ventricle and into the pulmonary artery, where it is wedged into a small branch. In that position, with the small branch of the artery plugged by the catheter, the tip of the catheter is actually recording the same pressure as in the left atrium, or the left ventricular filling pressure.

What Willie Ganz had developed was a catheter with a balloon on the end. After the catheter had been inserted into a vein, the balloon was inflated with air. The catheter then floated in the blood stream which carried it into the right atrium, the right ventricle, the pulmonary artery, and then down the pulmonary artery to a small branch. At this point the balloon could be deflated so it could measure the pressure in the pulmonary artery. The balloon would then be transiently re-inflated, thus occluding that small branch of the pulmonary artery and recording a pressure that we call left ventricular filling pressure.

Willie came to the Washington V.A. Hospital to display his invention before he published his first report. I was fascinated by what appeared to be the simplicity of performing this catheterization blindly at the bedside, but I was skeptical as to whether physicians would be willing to use such a catheter and inflate a balloon floating in the circulatory system of their patients. I told Willie that the method was interesting but unlikely to be clinically appealing.

How wrong I was! Within a few years after introduction of this balloon flotation catheter it became standard therapy in the management of acutely ill patients with severe cardiac dysfunction around the world. But in the early 1970s, this methodology was just becoming popular. We decided that it might serve as a practical means of recording left ventricular filling pressure at the bedside of our patients.

For us to document and monitor LV filling pressure, all patients in the trial would need to have a balloon flotation catheter placed in the pulmonary artery. This catheter would need to be left in place for the duration of the infusion. We made the decision, largely on the basis of what we thought might be desirable and achievable, that the infusion would be given for 48 hours. The goal, therefore, was to provide a 48-hour infusion of either nitroprusside or a sugar water solution (given double-blind) in patients who were still having chest pain from an AMI or were within 24 hours of the cessation of chest pain. We decided that our goal should be to reduce mortality, which is what is referred to as a "hard" endpoint, since there is no controversy about its occurrence.

What would be an appropriate follow-up time? It had to be the same for every patient entered into the trial. We didn't want to make it too short, since an improvement in heart function should have a long-term benefit. We didn't want to make it too long, since follow-up is complicated and these patients might be susceptible to other problems that could influence their life expectancy. We compromised on a 90-day follow-up, so our end-point for the study was 90-day mortality from all causes. Of course, that means deaths from non-cardiac causes, even automobile accidents, will count—but in the first three months after a heart attack, the vast majority of deaths are related to the heart attack. Furthermore, it is often difficult to know the immediate cause of death in individual patients.

Our biostatistical colleague was charged with calculating a sample size that would give us adequate power to detect a favorable effect of the therapy on this outcome. To do this we needed to predict the mortality rate at 90 days for this population, and the level of nitroprusside benefit we would like to detect. We concluded that we would need 1000 patients. I calculated that we should be able to recruit about 90 patients from each center. Therefore, we would need 11 participating centers to conduct the trial. The Cooperative Studies program approved our plans and budget, and I set out to recruit colleagues in various V.A. centers.

Little did my colleagues know that their decision to participate in this clinical trial would lead to a long-term collaboration involving several subsequent trials that would dramatically influence not only the field of cardiology, but also their individual research careers.

A fundamental flaw in our planning for this new, remarkably ambitious trial was that we did not assign it an acronym. It was early in the history of clinical trials, and acronyms had not yet become commonplace. I was somewhat intolerant of the use of clever acronyms, which often seemed like a manipulative effort to invent a title for a trial. Such titles as MR. FIT (Multiple Risk Factor Intervention Trial), CONSENSUS (Cooperative North Scandinavian Enalapril Survival Study) and SOLVD (Studies of Left Ventricular Dysfunction) have subsequently become part of the lexicon of clinical trials and are recognized by everyone who is interested in the field. We didn't select a catchy acronym for our trial, and thus it probably never achieved the degree of visibility that it otherwise deserved.

Go west young man

During the planning phase of this trial in 1975, I had left the V.A. in Washington, D.C. and moved to Minneapolis as Head of the Cardiovascular Division at the University of Minnesota. The decision to move was not reached lightly. My research productivity in Washington had not been limited by burdensome service and administrative responsibilities. I had carved out my own program, aided by enthusiastic junior trainees, most of them foreign medical graduates seeking to establish academic careers in their home countries or in the United Sates. The V.A. had provided a remarkable environment for the performance of clinical research.

But there were limitations to the growth of my program in Washington. I could not recruit colleagues, since I had no permanent positions to fill. I was a lone member of my own Division: Hypertension and Clinical Hemodynamics. Georgetown, my academic home, was not a progressive school and did not have an active research program. I had no restrictions on my personal activity, but I had no prospects for the growth of my program.

The position in Minnesota had many attractions. It was a large and vibrant university with a great tradition of clinical research. The city was attractive, exciting, and offered a remarkable quality of life. And I would now have a large Division and the opportunity to recruit young faculty to join me in our endeavors.

I was aware of the risks. My time would now be occupied with administrative and clinical duties. Recruitment is time-consuming and often frustrating. Furthermore, I would be taking on responsibility for a cardiology program even though my only specific cardiology training was a result of catheterizing the left ventricle. Would I be able to pull it off?

A big issue was my motive in accepting the position. In years to come I often warned young faculty members who sought my advice to "never take a job bigger than you are". By that I meant the job shouldn't be the determinant of who you are, because if it is you will be painfully diminished if you lose the job. The job should provide an opportunity for your growth, not serve as a badge of your accomplishment. That is how I viewed the position in Minnesota.

Fortunately, my family supported the move. Our three teenage children were excited about the adventure. Syma was reluctant to leave our beautiful new house in the Maryland suburbs of Washington, and hesitant about being separated from the University of Maryland campus where she was involved in writing a thesis for her master's degree in Art History. But she, too, felt that Minnesota would provide opportunities for the whole family not immediately available in Washington.

The V.A. staff had a going-away party for us and presented us with cross-country skis, a seemingly appropriate but somewhat ominous foreboding of life in Minnesota. We used them twice during our first winter in Minneapolis, and then stored them in a remote part of the garage. For us, winter was the season to spend indoors.

The uniqueness of Minneapolis became apparent soon after we settled into our newly-purchased home at the south end of Lake Harriet. On a beautiful sunny afternoon, we took our first walk around the lake, a three-mile trek that became a regular exercise route. The people we passed were mostly tall and blonde. As we passed, they invariably smiled and said hello. The motto "Minnesota Nice" was well deserved.

Since Minneapolis had a very active V.A. hospital, I accepted a part-time appointment at the V.A. so I could continue my V.A.-supported research activities while based at the University several miles away. The V.A. gave me permission to move all of our hemodynamic monitoring equipment from the Washington V.A. to the Minneapolis V.A. I brought a colleague with me from the Washington V.A. to head up research in the Minneapolis V.A., and Joe Franciosa became an important collaborator in our subsequent work. I also hired a V.A. research nurse who became a key contributor to our clinical research program. Susan Ziesche was appointed as the overall nurse coordinator for our nitroprusside trial. Her dedication to excellence, her bulldog determination, and her untiring perseverance were critical to maintaining the demanding protocol in our collaborating centers. She became the mother-figure and mentor of all of the nurses working in the program.

We deliver the drug

There had been no prior experience with a protocol such as our nitroprusside study in patients with an acute myocardial infarction. Never had so many infarct patients had their hearts catheterized to document pressure measurements. Recruitment for study patients was a major undertaking since we had to identify potential candidates as soon as possible after admission. Hospitalization for AMI occurs at all times of the day and night. The investigator and the local study coordinator needed to be on call around-the-clock if they were to be successful in recruitment. Furthermore, patients had to give informed consent to be screened for participation in the study, and the screening included catheterization of the heart with a balloon-tipped catheter. Patients in the hours after sustaining an AMI are stressed, often sedated by narcotics and not always able to provide proper informed consent. Family members were usually asked to participate in the consent process, but they were often also under stress. It is hardly surprising that overall recruitment was slow. Some centers were remarkably productive, and others were more effective in providing excuses for poor recruitment. Susan Ziesche spent hours on the phone with these Centers to encourage greater effort.

Once patients were recruited and had signed informed consent, the work began. The catheter was inserted from an arm vein into the heart with the aid of Willie Ganz's floating balloon tip. If the pressure elevation was high enough to meet the entrance criterion, and if no other complications rendered the patient ineligible, a sealed envelope was opened to identify the coded medication that was to be administered to the patient. The local investigator had no way to know whether the colored vials of medication were nitroprusside or placebo. The protocol mandated that the infusion had to be initiated within one hour after opening the envelope. This meant the medication in the vial had to be placed into a plastic bag of sugar water that was carefully wrapped with aluminum foil to protect it from light, which decomposes nitroprusside.

Over the next hour or two, the infusion rate for a patient was gradually increased to an established maximum level until either the LV filling pressure fell by 60%, or the infusion rate could not be increased because of a fall in blood pressure below a critical level, or because of other side effects. Once the infusion rate had been stabilized, it was the research team's responsibility to see that the infusion was continued for 48 hours. Needless to say, the demands on the investigator and the study nurse for each patient were considerable.

The trial took over five years to complete. During these years we had periodic meetings of the investigators and the nurse coordinators from each center, so camaraderie developed within the study team. Most of the gatherings were held in Minneapolis, and the party at our home became a regular event. The first couple of parties maintained a certain decorum as everyone got to know each other. But by the third year things began to get out of hand. It probably wasn't helped much by my whiskey sour concoction that everyone thought tasted like a simple punch. By the end of the evening people were sliding down the banister from the second floor and some of the nurses and investigators were found in compromising positions in various areas of the house. Syma ruled that it was the last party to be held at our house. We subsequently went to restaurants when the group gathered.

As in all prospective, randomized trials, it was critical that neither the investigators nor the patients knew whether the active treatment (in this case nitroprusside) or the placebo was administered to individual patients. Although the packets of drug were carefully blinded, and randomization was by selection of a sealed envelope, skeptics insisted that it would be impossible to blind the use of sugar water versus a drug that reliably lowers blood pressure and LV filling pressure. Certainly the nurses and doctors will know immediately whether they are giving the active drug or placebo, they claimed. And this knowledge might alter their approach to the patient and destroy the integrity of a blinded comparison between the two treatments.

We didn't want to fall into the same trap that doomed Irving Wright in his trial of warfarin. So we conducted a little sub-study. At the end of the infusion period the nurse-coordinators and physicians were asked to check a box as to whether they thought the patient had received nitroprusside or placebo. To our surprise and relief, after completion of the trial, we found that 30% of the time they had guessed wrong. Amazingly, given the variability of pressure measurements and of the response to the drug, our blinding was pretty well maintained and the integrity of the study was not compromised.

Study data were collected at the V.A. Cooperative Studies Coordinating Center in West Haven, CT. Overseeing the accumulating results was an Operations Committee (now usually called a Data Safety and Monitoring Committee). I appointed the members of this Operations Committee from expert colleagues at medical schools not involved in the study. The Operations Committee met every six months to review results and make certain the patients entered into the trial were not being harmed. These committees really act as patient advocates.

Although the biostatistician collecting the data in West Haven held the code that allowed him to know who had been given the study drug, he provided data to the Committee in blinded form, "Treatment A" and "Treatment B". The Committee was empowered to decide whether to review the data either without knowing which was the active treatment group or to break the blind. In any case, the data, whether blinded or unblinded, were seen only by the study biostatistician and members of the Committee, and all copies were destroyed after the meeting. As Study Chairman I never saw the data, but I met with the Committee at each meeting. I urged them to remain blinded. My rationale was that since nitroprusside was available and widely used, it was equally important to know if it was beneficial or harmful in AMI. Breaking the blind would only be helpful if one were likely to make a different decision based on whether Treatment A or Treatment B was exhibiting a more favorable effect. In my view, unblinding the data could wait until the trial was completed.

The Committee agreed.

We analyze the results

In January 1981, we terminated further entry into the protocol after 812 patients had been randomized. We had catheterized over 1600 patients with AMI, but many turned out to be ineligible because their filling pressures were too low. Our goal to study 1000 patients was not met, but we had the largest study—and certainly the most complex—ever undertaken in such acutely ill patients.

Our hypothesis had been that unrecognized failure of the left ventricle in AMI was contributing to worsening damage to the heart, and that relieving it with nitroprusside infusion in the early hours after the event would favorably affect prognosis. We recognized that the first 24 hours after an AMI is a volatile period, and that there is great variability from patient to patient in the severity of the heart damage and the patient's response.

When we examined the data in the 812 patients entered in the trial we were elated about the effectiveness of nitroprusside to control the heart failure. In the 407 patients given the active drug, nitroprusside, the LV filling pressure fell promptly from an average of 20 mmHg to 12 mmHg. It remained at that level for the entire duration of the infusion (Figure V-2). That average reduction of eight mmHg, we reasoned, should have resulted in improved blood supply to the inner layer of heart muscle and therefore could have reduced the extent of the muscle damage. In the 405 patients in the control group, however, LV filling pressure fell gradually. After 48 hours it was at a level similar to that in the treated group. The issue, then, was whether this 48 hours of protecting the inner layer of heart would favorably affect outcome.

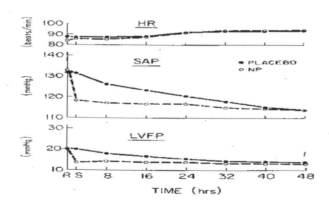

Figure V-2

The mean changes observed during 48 hours of drug infusions in 812 patients entered into the nitroprusside trial. The left ventricular filling pressure (LVFP) and the systolic arterial pressure (SAP) fell promptly in response to nitroprusside but fell gradually in response to the placebo infusion. Heart rate was not affected by nitroprusside.

We also had collected sequential blood samples from all the patients to measure the amount of an enzyme (creatine kinase MB) released from damaged heart muscle into the blood stream. Heart muscle cells, or myocytes, contain a number of specific substances that are thought to be released only when the cell dies and the cell wall ruptures. This measurement of the amount of CKMB appearing in the blood had become accepted as a measure of "infarct size"—the amount of heart muscle damaged by the attack. We discovered that the patients treated with nitroprusside released less enzyme than those treated with placebo, apparently confirming a favorable effect of nitroprusside on heart muscle damage.

Our joy dissipated when we first looked at the outcome data. The death rate in the two groups was quite similar. By 21 days, about 11% of each group had died, and by three months the mortality in the nitroprusside group was 17% and in the placebo group 19%, a difference that was not statistically significant. Clearly, AMI was a serious disease with a high mortality. Unfortunately, our treatment was not adequate to change its course. After five years of Herculean effort, we had failed to show a significant benefit of nitroprusside infusion despite its favorable effects on heart function and an apparently favorable effect on heart muscle damage.

What had happened? Why didn't this benefit on function and damage translate into improved outcome? By three months, nearly 20% of the patients had died. Why hadn't nitroprusside reduced their risk of dying? What characterized the 20% who had died versus the 80% who had survived?

We were seeking a new understanding about what happens after an acute MI. It would eventually explain the mechanism of Sam Farber's course and of all the new treatments for heart failure yet to be developed. But in 1981 we were still limited by what we could measure. We could measure function of the left ventricle with our balloon catheter. We could measure pressure and heart muscle damage. We could certainly identify who lives and who dies. But we did not yet have imaging techniques that would allow us to visualize heart structures in unstable, acutely ill patients. We could monitor function but not structure.

As we examined our outcome data more carefully, a remarkable pattern emerged. The effectiveness of nitroprusside was critically dependent on the interval between the initial pain of the heart attack and the initiation of infusion of the drug. The pattern was so consistent and dramatic that the *New England Journal of Medicine*, the bastion of medical conservatism, agreed to publish our manuscript with the time-dependent subgroup outcome as the major feature of the paper. Normally, when the primary end-point of a trial is negative, as it was in our trial, no subgroup analysis is allowed except to explore possible strategies for a new study. But in this case the subgroup analysis turned a negative trial into a positive trial.

What we had found was that those patients whose elevated LV filling pressures were detected and nitroprusside infusion started within nine hours of the onset of their pain did less well on nitroprusside than on placebo. Most of these patients probably had only modest damage to their hearts and would have recovered spontaneously in the next few hours, just as many of our patients did when we first began monitoring their LV filling pressure. They weren't really in heart failure. They merely had a transient increase in filling pressure as a consequence of the myocardial infarction. Treatment to interfere with their normal defense mechanisms by relaxing their arteries and lowering their blood pressure could only harm them, not help them.

Sam Farber had certainly not been in this group.

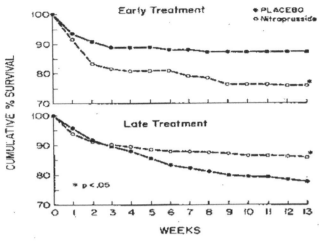

Figure V-3

Survival over 13 weeks in patients entered into the nitroprusside trial. In those in whom infusions were begun within nine hours of the onset of their heart attack pain (early treatment) nitroprusside appeared to reduce survival, whereas in those entered later nitroprusside appeared to have a delayed benefit on survival, the difference from the placebo survival appearing after about four weeks

In stark contrast was the response in patients screened and treated more than nine hours after the onset of the event. Their elevated filling pressure obviously had persisted. They undoubtedly had suffered more heart muscle damage, and most of them were probably destined to develop persistent heart failure because of that damage. Sam Farber was certainly one of these patients.

In those patients who received the placebo, 22% of them died within three months, whereas in those given nitroprusside the mortality rate was only 14%, a statistically significant benefit on outcome. Nitroprusside had clearly slowed or halted a process likely to progress. That process had to have something to do with heart failure, which had led to Sam Farber's death. And that process would eventually reveal itself as a structural change, something we were unable to measure routinely in

1980. This structural change would eventually gain the label of "ventricular remodeling".

Our No-Name trial was a tremendous learning experience for us all. We showed that complex and demanding multicenter trials could be carried out if you had a dedicated group of investigators. Patients could be recruited into such trials, but more centers would be needed to recruit adequate patients in a reasonable time. We learned that having an acronym for a trial guarantees more long-term recognition. In addition, analysis and publication of all the ancillary data from a trial this complex would have required more support for data analysis than the V.A. was willing to provide.

As part of the No-Name protocol, we had collected a host of important short-term and long-term information that never saw the light of day. The investigators all became too busy doing new things, including new studies that we initiated. The Cooperative Studies Data Support Center personnel were assigned to other projects as soon as our primary manuscript was published. Potentially important observations were never fully analyzed and important papers were never written. This reduced the potential impact of the study. I vowed never to let that happen again.

My thoughts were also racing forward beyond the syndrome of acute MI.

If short-term infusion of nitroprusside was effective in altering the course of patients who had persistent acute heart failure after an AMI, would it be effective in patients with chronic heart failure? Our hospitals were full of patients with heart failure. It was and still is the leading cause of hospitalization in the Medicare population. My interests were about to shift to the chronic disease process called heart failure.

CHAPTER VI
Heart Failure

By the time our No-Name trial was completed in 1981 I had already been in Minnesota for seven years. The trial was based at the V.A. Hospital, which was almost 10 miles from my office and my responsibilities at the University of Minnesota. Most of my waking hours were devoted not to the trial, but to my effort to build a strong academic program at the University. Syma was thriving in the Minneapolis art and literary community and our three children were all off to college in New England, never having fully shed their East Coast roots. Even our cat, Frizz, had died, leaving us free of responsibilities at home, except for our all-too-big house in the block just south of a city lake.

The University's Cardiovascular Division, which it was now called, consisted of four independent hospitals—the University Hospital, the V.A. Hospital, the Hennepin County Hospital in Minneapolis, and the Ramsey County Hospital in St. Paul. Each of these had University faculty dedicated to patient care and, I hoped, research and teaching. I had responsibility for aiding in recruitment and for the performance of the faculty at all hospitals, but my primary dedication was to the core faculty at the University Hospital. The hospital was small and dedicated to tertiary care—dealing with complex problems that the private hospitals in the community were not prepared to handle. When I arrived, the faculty was composed predominantly of older physicians not active in research. My first goal was recruitment, and I succeeded in attracting a number of future academic leaders in the subspecialties of cardiology.

We also convinced outstanding trainees to choose Minnesota as the site for their education. Many of these remained in the Twin Cities to enhance both the academic and practice community.

All of this activity demanded a dedicated administrative staff to support the faculty, trainees and programs. My choice of an administrator was a key to our future success. Cheryl Yano brought to the program incredible talent, dedication and productivity that impacted everyone in the Division. After I stepped down as division director in 1996, I recruited her to become Executive Director of the Heart Failure Society of America, an organization I founded in 1995 and that became the societal home for all American doctors and scientists specializing in the study of heart failure and its clinical care. Equally important to my personal stability was a talented and dedicated administrative assistant, Nina Lacis, whose judgment, maturity and efficiency made it possible for me to pursue my objectives for the program while juggling all my other activities.

The focus of my attention

Fascination with heart failure is what drove me into cardiology and brought me to Minnesota. Acute myocardial infarction is a form of acute heart failure that may persist and worsen, as it did with Sam Farber. In some patients with this form of acute heart failure, however, the failure recovers after a few days, as documented in our No- Name trial.

Chronic heart failure was different. It was viewed as an established abnormality in the function of the heart that persisted and worsened. It was the most common cause of hospitalization in the Medicare population of America. It burdened our hospitals and our health care system. And we had no effective means of slowing its progression and restoring patients to an active life. My experience with heart failure in Washington convinced me that it should be the focus of my attention when I assumed the cardiology post at the University of Minnesota.

All medical students learn about heart failure early in their medical school curriculum. It was traditionally called "congestive heart failure"—CHF for short. It has been known over the years as a chronic disease, usually of the elderly, that represents the ultimate common pathway of progression of all forms of heart disease. It causes fluid accumulation or congestion in the lungs and swelling of the ankles, and results from weakening of the pumping ability of the heart leading inexorably to reduced exercise tolerance and premature death. In the 1960s, two treatments were known: 1) diuretics, which worked by ridding the body of the extra fluid by an action on the kidneys; and 2) digitalis, a product of the leaves of the foxglove plant that increased the force of heart contraction and slowed heart rate. But the disease, students were told, was progressive. Everyone who had it would eventually die from it.

During the summer of my first year in medical school I worked on a project with my uncle, Harry Gold, who was introduced in Chapter IV when he ministered to my mother after her heart attack. Harry was not only a practicing cardiologist but was also a professor of pharmacology at Cornell. He was well known for his work in isolated heart preparations to show that digitalis increases the strength of muscle contraction of the failing heart by making heart muscle contract more vigorously. Uncle Harry was one of the first clinical trialists, an advocate for studying drugs in carefully designed "blinded" trials.

My uncle was famous as a story teller. He recounted to my second-year class the story of a new drug he was testing for angina, the chest pain caused by coronary artery blockages that interfere with blood flow to nourish the heart muscle. He had designed a cross-over trial, one in which patients were blindly assigned to an investigational drug or a matching placebo for a period of time to assess the effects, hopefully to show that the new drug was superior to the placebo pill. Then the patients were reassigned to the opposite therapy for a similar interval—thus a "cross-over" study. Neither the patients nor the care providers were allowed to know which pill they were taking at any given time. In Harry's study, he found several patients who exhibited a dramatically favorable response to the treatment. His investigative team was excited about what they assumed was a beneficial effect of their experimental therapy. When the code was broken, however, the favorable responses were more common with the placebo. The active drug obviously did not work.

Harry's point, of course, was to convince the class that placebo-controlled trials were critical to establish the benefit of a new therapy. Apparently favorable responses to placebo are generally viewed as indicative of the variability of disease symptoms.

Medical lore tells the story of a famous, megomaniacal surgeon who was a visiting lecturer at a medical school. He had developed a surgical procedure to treat a particularly difficult disease. After presenting his data, a medical student raised his hand and asked if the surgeon had considered doing a controlled trial, in which half the patients selected for the procedure were randomly assigned not to get it in order to demonstrate that the procedure led to a favorable outcome. The surgeon boomed in response: "What? And doom half the patients to certain death?" To which the student quietly asked, "Which half?"

I had been assigned by my uncle in 1957 to study the effects of a diuretic, mercuhydrin, in patients with heart failure. The drug was known to enhance sodium and water excretion by the kidney, thus hopefully ridding the body of the excess fluid or edema. It was a powerful diuretic. Since the drug had to be administered by intramuscular injection, the patients came in every other day for an injection. I did not know if any particular injection was mercuhydrin or harmless sugar-water. I was "blinded", and so was the patient, thus the term "double-blind". At the end of the summer we broke the code and analyzed the results, which showed that the mercuhydrin had produced dramatic weight loss and improvement in shortness of breath and ankle edema.

Harry was so impressed by the results of our little trial that he excitedly began to advocate changing the name of "congestive heart failure" to "congestive failure" to reflect his growing view that the kidney, not the heart, was the organ at fault, and that the word "heart" could appropriately be removed from the definition. It was only years later, when it was demonstrated that transplanting a new heart into a patient with CHF reversed the disease, that we could comfortably claim that the heart was certainly the culprit. It is ironic that nearly 40 years after my uncle tried to change "congestive heart failure" to "congestive failure" I advocated changing the name from "congestive heart failure" to "heart failure", thus acknowledging the growing evidence that the heart could fail and kill people without the patient necessarily manifesting "congestion" or swelling. (In the past year I have had a medical journal dialogue with a critic who is clamoring for elimination of the word "failure" in the name because it is too depressing to patients. Semantic arguments may never cease.)

What causes heart failure?

The most common cause of heart failure in the 1950s and 1960s was longstanding hypertension. It still is a common factor, but two changes in health care have resulted in a major alteration in the prevalence of heart failure causes. Better treatment of hypertension means that blood pressure is lower these days and therefore imposes less of a chronic burden on the heart to cause it to fail. In addition, chronic damage to heart muscle initially from a heart attack (Acute Myocardial Infarction, See Chapter IV) has become a more common cause of heart failure, largely because the in-hospital mortality from myocardial infarction has fallen from 20% to 5%, thus sending many more patients home with heart muscle damage likely to lead years later to heart failure.

We didn't always know why patients developed heart failure, which was common in elderly patients, often without any apparent precipitating cause. Some young people also developed it without any clearcut cause. The term cardiomyopathy emerged to provide doctors with a diagnostic term. All it means is that something is wrong with the heart (cardio) muscle (myopathy). The term needs a modifier for explanation. "Hypertensive" was added when the patient had a long history of hypertension. "Ischemic", meaning inadequate blood flow to nourish the muscle, was added when the apparent cause was a previous MI. "Alcoholic" was added in heavy drinkers because we learned that excess alcohol consumption can damage heart muscle in some individuals. In many individuals the term "Idiopathic" was added because we had no explanation, and that's what the word means.

In the 1960s, the conventional wisdom was that chronic hypertension caused heart failure by burdening the left ventricle so that it eventually failed as a pump. That means either that the amount of blood pumped by the heart into the tissues of the body was inadequate to support the demands of the body for blood flow; or, alternatively, that the only way the heart could pump enough blood to serve the body's needs was by a stretching of the chamber to increase its force of contraction.

Based on the Frank-Starling curve shown earlier (Figure III-3), the depression of the function curve of the left ventricle means that either the output is too low or the filling pressure too high. Either one of these abnormalities will lead to symptoms such as fatigue, reduced exercise tolerance, and shortness of breath. Because of the backup of fluid behind the heart, there is often congestion in the lungs and swelling of the ankles. These are the classical signs and symptoms of heart failure.

The impedance curves shown in Figure III-5 raised another possibility. Could heightened impedance produce a force that opposed emptying of the left ventricle when it contracts? Could this increased resistance to blood ejection be adversely affecting heart function in patients with chronic heart failure even if their blood pressure is not elevated? Would a vasodilator drug, by lowering impedance, improve heart function in a patient with severe heart failure that hadn't responded to standard treatment?

In 1973, at the Washington V.A. Hospital, we had the drug—sodium nitroprusside. And we had the tools to monitor response. All we needed was a patient.

Experimenting on a patient

It did not take long to test the hypothesis. Many patients with severe heart failure were hospitalized for management of their condition. At that point most of them had low blood pressure, not high blood pressure, presumably because the heart could no longer pump enough blood to keep their pressure up. They were given digoxin, diuretics, and tender loving care because everyone recognized that this was an end-stage disease. The patients were not expected to live long.

Our first volunteer was an ideal candidate. He was a 68-year-old man who had suffered two previous heart attacks. Harold Campbell had a younger wife (his second) and four apparently devoted children who were at his bedside when I visited. His heart failure had progressively worsened over the previous six months, and his family described his gradual decline in ability to walk and his breathing difficulty while lying down. He had been hospitalized for 10 days in an attempt to rid his body of excess fluid. He was being treated with digoxin and a potent diuretic that was being given intravenously to squeeze more fluid out through his kidney. The therapy was not working and he was weak, short of breath, and had marked swelling of his feet and legs.

After explaining the plan to Harold and his family, I summoned my team and shooed the family out of the room. We performed our usual bedside catheterization. His arterial pressure was 126/84 mmHg (normal), his left ventricular filling pressure was 35 mmHg (very high), and his cardiac output was very low. Despite normal blood pressure, therefore, the resistance and impedance of his circulation was very high (See Figure III-5) and his heart had weakened. Constricted blood vessels were maintaining his blood pressure despite the markedly reduced blood flow. We cautiously initiated an infusion of sodium nitroprusside.

To our amazement and satisfaction, as the dose was gradually increased, his LV filling pressure fell and his cardiac output rose with little effect on his blood pressure. We had reduced impedance without lowering blood pressure.

Remember that blood pressure is the product of cardiac output and peripheral resistance (Figure I-1). If resistance is decreased and output is comparably increased, blood pressure need not change. Heart function, however, would be much better.

Harold's breathing improved and his urine output increased briskly. "I haven't been able to breathe so easily for six months," Harold reported. We had relieved his severe heart failure not by stimulating the heart, but rather by reducing the impedance load against which it was pumping. We had theorized—and now demonstrated—that impedance could be a critical determinant of cardiac function in chronic heart failure, even when the blood pressure is normal (Figure III-5).

It's hard to describe the elation I felt in the hours after this experience. Not only had my theory been proved correct, but we had introduced a new and remarkably effective therapy for heart failure. Patients dying from progressive heart failure could now be helped by an entirely new approach to treatment. I wanted to tell the world and hasten the delivery of this therapy to the thousands and perhaps millions of patients worldwide suffering from this often terminal condition. But by the next day I realized that prudence required that our observation should be confirmed before it was celebrated.

Harold Campbell was an anecdote. We had to demonstrate that his response to nitroprusside was not a fluke. We began a search for other patients hospitalized with severe and poorly responding chronic heart failure. They were not hard to find. After a few months we had accumulated experience with 18 patients from the wards of the Washington V.A. Hospital. They were all men who ranged in age from 33 to 81 years old. Women were a rarity in V.A. hospitals in the 1970s. Nine of the patients had previously suffered from an MI, so they fit the diagnosis of ischemic cardiomyopathy. The other nine had no such history and were labeled as idiopathic cardiomyopathy. All of them were suffering from severe heart failure despite treatment with digoxin and diuretic. In response to nitroprusside infusion their symptoms were relieved, their cardiac output rose, their filling pressure fell, and their urine output increased. Kidney function improved dramatically. All of this happened with only a slight fall in blood pressure.

A new era

This time the *New England Journal of Medicine* promptly accepted our manuscript and published it as the lead article on September 19,

1974. Either their editorial board had become less stodgy or they now viewed intervention in this chronic condition less potentially dangerous than in heart failure accompanying an acute MI. For years after, and even still today, young and now older cardiologists stop me at meetings to tell me that it was this paper that enticed them into their cardiology careers.

This paper changed forever our approach to the management of heart failure. It represented the birth of vasodilator therapy for heart failure and, with it, a lesson on the physiology of the linkage between the heart and the blood vessels that had previously been unrecognized.

Why had no one previously appreciated this response to vasodilators and recommended it as a therapy? How could such a prominent effect have not been appreciated before? I searched the literature and found only sporadic reports suggesting that perhaps the idea had been considered in years past but never formally tested.

I remembered, somewhat troublingly, an experience in 1965 when, as chairman of the local section of the American Federation for Clinical Research (AFCR), I moderated a series of research presentations at our annual meeting in Washington, D.C. One young author reported on a dog model of shock with a very low cardiac output. He had infused a drug that relaxed the arteries and noted a marked rise in cardiac output. He had provided no rational explanation for this observation, but claimed that the drug led to an improvement in cardiac function. As a confident young clinical physiologist who thought he understood the principles of left ventricular function, I had patiently explained to him—probably in an unfortunately pedantic style, that this improvement in function could only be explained by an effect of the drug to increase contractility by an inotropic effect on the heart. It must, I had opined, directly stimulate the heart.

I was wrong. This was an experimental observation that pre-dated mine but was never pursued. In the 1960s, heart function was defined by Frank-Starling curves that identified a favorable shift of the curve as an inotropic effect (Figure III-3). It was only after our studies in hy-

pertensive heart failure that we could identify an independent role of
pressure or impedance in defining cardiac function (Figure III-5). We
had reaffirmed that in patients with an acute MI. We now had expanded
that concept to include patients with chronic heart failure and normal or
even low blood pressures.

So our observation of the favorable effect of vasodilators may not
have been new, but it had remained unknown to the medical community.

In retrospect, it should have been obvious. All pumps have a limit
to the pressure they can pump against. The heart is no exception. If one
obstructs the aorta—the main artery into which the heart empties—the
heart must generate a higher pressure to eject blood. If the pressure requirement is high enough, the heart will fail. So in unusual experimental
situations it had always been clear that the heart's function could be
influenced by outflow resistance or impedance.

But in the physiologic range of pressure and resistance, the heart
seemed to miraculously adjust its performance to match the required
work, that remarkable phenomenon previously described as "autoregulation". This mechanism was adequate to maintain normal output from
the heart in the face of striking changes in resistance and pressure. So
the outflow resistance to the pump's emptying was never felt to be an
important factor in determining heart function. It was only in the damaged heart that we identified this striking dependence on resistance to
outflow from the heart. This resistance was increased by the heightened
tone of the arteries, which could be relaxed by nitroprusside and (presumably) by the blocking agent utilized in dogs by that unnamed young
investigator in 1965.

I was ready to publicize more widely my new approach to treatment.
Circulation, the prestigious journal of the American Heart Association,
published my submitted editorial announcing this new concept: "Vasodilator therapy for heart failure: The role of impedance on left ventricular function." A prominent medical journal invited me to organize a
symposium in their pages discussing this new linking of the heart and
the blood vessels. I entitled it "Marriage of the Heart and the Circula-

tion" and described it as a "shotgun wedding" because of the traditional isolation of these specialists.

Another surprising thing happened. We had purchased the nitroprusside that we used in our studies from a chemical company as a powder, and then prepared it in my own laboratory for intravenous use. It was not commercially available. We had described the method for its preparation and sterilization in our publications, and other hospitals around the country had begun preparing and using it. There was no national restriction on such use as long as it did not cross state borders.

The Food and Drug Administration became appropriately concerned. In the absence of strict standards for preparation, they could not countenance its widespread use. The director of the FDA approached Hoffman la Roche, which was providing the chemical powder to us, and asked if they would be willing to market it as a drug.

This must have been a first— the FDA asking a company to market a drug. The FDA made an unusual offer to Hoffman la Roche. If the company would review my patient records and submit an application for approval based on our data, the FDA would approve the drug for marketing.

I was naïve. As an academic I didn't think about financial gain from my research. We had made the discovery of the effectiveness of nitroprusside, but since it was an old chemical I was unaware that I could have patented this new and original use, even if the drug was generic. Only years later did I learn of "Use Patents". Because of this naiveté, I gave Hoffman la Roche free access to my files and asked for nothing in return. The company submitted an application to the FDA with the support of 15 patient studies. The drug was approved without further study and subsequently marketed as "Nipride". It is still widely used in intensive care units around the world. I don't want to know how much money I lost by not making a licensing deal with the company, now Roche Pharmaceuticals. But I did learn never to miss an opportunity like that again.

This new integration of the heart with the vasculature had implications beyond improved management for the failing heart. It meant that cardiologists who had focused exclusively on the heart as if it were an isolated organ now had to pay attention to the blood vessels. For many traditional, old-school cardiologists, this was difficult to accept. Integrative physiology, which attempted to understand the circulation and its multiple neural, hormonal, vascular and cardiac influences, was outside the expertise of these classically trained clinicians who focused on heart sounds with ever-improving acoustical stethoscopes. They interpreted electrocardiograms, the electrical signals that control the heart rhythm and help define the route of the electrical impulse throughout the muscle. But they were not comfortable with determinants of blood pressure, the role of hormones on the blood vessels and heart, the complex circulatory adjustments during exercise, etc. So for many of those traditional cardiologists, the marriage between the heart and circulation was at the end of a "shotgun". And for the vascular doctors, primarily interested in hypertension, the heart was foreign territory.

But the time had come. The heart was no longer an isolated organ. It was part of an integrated system that linked all the organs together.

We were only at the beginning of this new understanding. Just as with AMI, demonstrating an acute improvement in heart function did not necessarily mean that this improvement could be sustained and that the patient would be symptomatically improved or live longer. We needed to go beyond nitroprusside, which could only be given intravenously, and develop an oral vasodilator that could be given chronically. We needed a randomized clinical trial, not with the short-term outcome we had selected in AMI, but with a long-term outcome suitable for patients with chronic heart failure. The biggest challenges lay ahead, and they would need to be addressed at the University of Minnesota.

CHAPTER VII
Oral Vasodilator Therapy

The benefit of nitroprusside (NP) infusion in patients with severe heart failure and acute myocardial infarction (AMI) established the principle that a vasodilator drug could improve the function of the heart. But it left untested whether chronic therapy could alter the course of the disease. I was excited about the possibility that progression of heart failure was a manifestation of a vicious circle set into motion by constriction of the arteries. The impedance increase would lead to a reduction of cardiac output, which would lead to more constriction and a further fall in cardiac output eventuating in progressive deterioration of heart function and end-stage heart failure (Figure VII-1). Interruption of that cycle might be possible by relaxing the arteries in order to reduce impedance—the load opposing heart emptying during contraction.

This hypothesis couldn't explain the initial impairment of heart function that made it sensitive to impedance. I was comfortable that I understood how damage to the heart muscle would lead to that impairment, but the progressive decline—the process that killed Sam Farber—could have been the result of a vicious circle of artery constriction that could have been reversed.

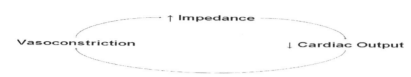

Figure VII – 1

When the function of the heart is impaired, it becomes sensitive to impedance, the total force in the blood vessels that opposes emptying of the left ventricle. Constriction of the small arteries raises impedance and leads to a fall in cardiac output.

Drugs like nitroprusside directly relax the arteries, so it may not matter why they are constricted. Whatever the cause, the drug should interfere with constriction. We were, however, seeking the *cause* of that constriction so we might deal with it more mechanistically. By identifying the cause of the constriction we might instead be able to use drugs that interfere with the processes that cause the arteries to constrict.

It was possible to explore a potential mechanism of this worsening constriction. Soon after arriving in Minnesota in 1974 I established a biochemistry research laboratory to serve our research program and hired a biochemist, Ada Simon. Ada, a native of Poland and a holocaust survivor, was a meticulous and dedicated scientist. She and her husband, Sidney, a professor of art history at the University, became good friends with whom Syma and I often socialized.

Do hormones play a role?

I suspected that hormone systems, known to be activated in heart failure, were contributing to the artery constriction. Methods for assessing blood levels of norepinephrine (secreted by the sympathetic nervous system), renin (secreted by the kidney) and vasopressin (secreted by the brain) were all available. All of these hormones were known to cause constriction of the arteries and a rise in blood pressure. Ada refined the methods in her laboratory.

In our initial studies, levels of these hormones all were higher in blood samples taken from patients with heart failure than they were in previously studied normal subjects, usually members of our research team. But I was concerned about the comparison. The patients with heart failure were different in age, background and life style from our staff. It occurred to me that a better comparator group would be the spouses of our patients, most of whom attended clinic visits with our patients. They were of similar age and background, and shared the same life style. Most were willing to offer their arm for obtaining a blood sample.

It turned out that levels of all these hormones were much higher in the patients with heart failure than in their spouses. So our hypothesis could comfortably be expanded to suggest that heart failure activated these hormonal systems, and the release of these hormones led to artery constriction, an increase of impedance, and the initiation of a vicious circle that resulted in progressive heart failure (Figure VII-2).

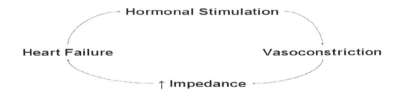

Figure VII – 2

Activation of the sympathetic nervous system and the renin-angiotensin system may be an important cause of the small artery vasoconstriction that raises impedance and leads to heart failure.

In order to test this hypothesis we needed to induce long-term relaxation of the arteries. We had two alternatives. We could relax the arteries by blocking the hormone systems that might be activating vasoconstriction, or we could administer a drug that directly relaxes or dilates the arteries—a vasodilator drug. The hypothesis was that this vascular effect, by whichever way we accomplished it, would slow progression of heart failure and relieve its symptoms.

Nitroprusside was not a practical option for long-term therapy. Not only did it require intravenous infusion, but prolonged administration led to the accumulation in the blood of toxic products, particularly thiocyanate. Consequently, prolonged infusions of nitroprusside required monitoring of thiocyanate levels so that the infusion could be discontinued before dangerous levels accumulated. We needed an oral therapy that could replicate the effects of nitroprusside and could be given chronically to patients with heart failure.

Nitroprusside in a pill

Not many available drugs fulfilled our criteria for vasodilators. In 1975, Joe Franciosa and I set about testing the available drugs in an effort to identify an agent that could produce the same effects as nitroprusside in patients with heart failure. We started with the nitrates. These were commonly used to treat patients with coronary artery disease because of their effect to relax the coronary artery and improve blood flow to the heart muscle. The mechanism of their action was not well understood, but it was known that a nitroglycerin tablet placed under the tongue would dissolve quickly and its absorption would abort an attack of angina or chest pain in a patient with coronary artery disease. The assumption was that the nitroglycerin improved the flow of blood through the coronary arteries to the myocardium and relieved ischemia, the imbalance between the demand of the heart muscle for oxygen and the ability of the coronary arteries to deliver that oxygen.

No one at that time fully understood how nitroglycerin relieved chest pain, but there was a rich literature describing the possible pathways by which a nitrate, nitroglycerin, administered under the tongue could improve the balance between blood flow and oxygen demand in the heart muscle. Since nitroprusside and nitroglycerin both harbored a nitrogen and an oxygen in their chemical structure, we suspected that their mode of action might be similar.

Only years later did the discovery of nitric oxide, a gas secreted by the inner lining of the blood vessel wall, lead to a Nobel Prize. And only with that discovery did we learn that nitroprusside and the nitrates all exert their effect by generating nitric oxide through their metabolic breakdown in the body.

We initially undertook studies with sublingual nitroglycerin, which dramatically lowered the LV filling pressure or pulmonary wedge pressure, but did not increase cardiac output, as did nitroprusside.

This observation was not surprising. The nitrates exert a powerful relaxing effect on veins but not much relaxing effect on the resistance arteries that control impedance. Dilation of the veins should lower the heart's filling pressure by allowing pooling of blood in the veins, thus reducing the flow back to the heart. But it would not be expected to increase the cardiac output because of the absence of much arterial relaxation or impedance reduction. Nitroprusside, on the other hand, exerts a powerful effect on both the arteries and the veins to reduce filling pressure and increase cardiac output.

To this day it is not fully understood why two drugs that enhance nitric oxide produce such different vascular effects.

A further problem was that the hemodynamic effect of sublingual nitroglycerin lasted less than 30 minutes and was therefore not a practical approach to chronic management. Oral nitrates were also available and widely used in clinical practice, although there was considerable controversy about whether they exerted much effect because of the presumed gastrointestinal destruction of the drug before it was absorbed. Nonetheless, we found that an orally administered drug called isosorbide dinitrate, marketed as Isordil or Sorbitrate, also lowered the LV filling pressure in patients with heart failure, and the effect lasted for four to six hours, making it a potentially useful for chronic therapy.

An ointment?

Nitroglycerin was also available as an ointment that was assumed to be absorbed through the skin. The history of the recognition of skin absorption is an interesting one. Munition workers in the 1940s were exposed to nitroglycerin, which served as an explosive. These workers suffered severe headaches, a common side effect of nitrates, when they began work at the beginning of the week, apparently as a result of skin absorption of the nitroglycerin. Later in the week the headaches would abate, presumably a consequence of tolerance that also was apparent in patients who took oral nitrates continuously. In fact, there was an unresolved issue as to whether the tolerance to headaches also meant tolerance to the blood vessel dilating effect of nitroglycerin.

The most fascinating phenomenon in these munition workers, however, was during the weekend when they were no longer in a nitroglycerin environment. They developed severe chest pain, as if their coronary arteries were undergoing spasm when the nitroglycerin was removed. They learned to smear some of the chemical on their skin during the weekend to prevent the chest pain.

Nitroglycerin was marketed as an ointment called Nitrol by a small pharmaceutical company, Kremers-Urban. The dose was measured in inches of the paste applied to the skin. We studied a few patients with heart failure who exhibited a fall in their left ventricular filling pressure that lasted at least four to six hours when the ointment was applied. I felt that the ointment deserved a more careful study and hoped that the company would fund it. I called them and received a visit from their vice-president, an elderly retired obstetrician who had joined the company a few years before.

I shared with him our excitement about the potential of Nitrol ointment as a treatment for heart failure. He had apparently become skeptical of the drug over the years because of the company's waning sales for the treatment of angina. He described their market research that revealed that the average age of the physicians prescribing Nitrol was 73 years old. He thought the market for the drug was ending. He was a most unusual company spokesperson! Most company officers are enthusiasts for their products. He was downright pessimistic.

I explained to him that this new potential use could revive the product. Then he revealed the true basis of his pessimism. The company he explained, had carried out studies of absorption. They had applied two inches to the skin, waited six hours, then removed the ointment. When they measured the nitroglycerin in two inches of the ointment and compared it to what was removed after six hours the amounts were identical. "The stuff isn't absorbed," he said.

They were not interested in funding a study.

I was skeptical of this report. We had seen a fall in pressure in the patients we had studied, even though it was not an adequately controlled trial. Were we possibly observing a placebo effect?

I came up with an idea. When it gets into the body, nitroglycerin causes headaches in normal people. Interestingly, it is much less likely to cause headaches in patients with heart disease. That distinction has long been known even though the mechanism of this difference is not well understood. I decided on a little experiment with my research group.

At the next staff meeting I asked each individual to allow the application of two inches of ointment on their arms. Everyone agreed and we sat down for our usual one-hour discussion. As I suspected, people got immersed in our business and forgot about the ointment.

After about 30 minutes, one of the technicians said "I've got a headache, and I never get headaches." Moments later, one of the nurses said "My head is throbbing." Then I too felt flushing and a dull headache. When we wiped off the ointment our symptoms abated. It was clear that Nitrol ointment was absorbed.

Despite Kremer-Urban's lack of support, however, transdermal nitroglycerin survived. We carried out a study in hypertensive patients whose blood pressures were inadequately controlled on two drugs. We added either Nitrol or a placebo ointment, double-blind, and found a significant fall in blood pressure over a 4-week study period. Other companies developed skin patches of nitroglycerin that released the drug in a more controlled way. These patches are still in widespread use for the treatment of angina. The absence of a market for the drug in hypertension reflects the fact that nitrates are generic and not a robust source of income for any manufacturer.

Hydralazine and isosorbide dinitrate

None of these nitrate preparations, we discovered, were effective in raising the cardiac output. Since one of the goals of vasodilator therapy was to improve output as well as to lower filling pressure, it was clear that we needed a different drug if we wanted to replicate the effects of nitroprusside.

Hydralazine was a vasodilator widely employed in those days to treat hypertension. Its effect was principally on the arteries and less on the veins. We anticipated that it would lower resistance to ejection without lowering the filling pressure very much.

Our studies with hydralazine confirmed this hypothesis. When we gave doses of 75 mg or greater to patients with heart failure, cardiac output increased dramatically, reflecting the lowering of resistance to left ventricular ejection. The major side effect was headache in some patients, but not in all. Since our goal was to both raise the cardiac output and lower the filling pressure, it seemed reasonable to combine the nitrate and the hydralazine.

We undertook a series of experiments with this drug combination, combining isosorbide dinitrate 20 mg and hydralazine 75 mg. Despite the effectiveness of the ointment, we decided it would be easier to control pill dosing than skin ointment dosing. We gave a group of heart failure patients an infusion of nitroprusside and observed a striking benefit on the function of the left ventricle. We then turned off the infusion and allowed the patients to return to their original state.

We then administered the two oral drugs and observed them for the next six hours. The response to the drug combination was identical to that of nitroprusside, and the effect lasted for up to six hours before beginning to wane. We had found an oral therapy that could reproduce the hemodynamic effects of nitroprusside. Furthermore, we grew optimistic about the long-term effects of isosorbide dinitrate used alone.

We already had a clinical experience.

The first clinical experiment

The year before leaving the Washington VA Hospital for Minneapolis I was confronted with a problem patient. Joseph Abbey was a 58-year-old postman who had suffered an acute myocardial infarction in another hospital six weeks earlier . After discharge, Mr. Abbey experienced gradually worsening shortness of breath and leg swelling. He was subsequently admitted to the VA Hospital with severe congestive heart failure. Despite aggressive attempts to relieve his congestion and improve the function of his heart, his condition deteriorated over the next few days. His course appeared to be similar to that of Sam Farber 17 years before.

On the fourth hospital day, he was drifting into shock with cool, clammy skin, marked congestion of his lungs and reduced urine output, symptoms identical to that of Sam Farber when he was readmitted with his terminal illness. We began an infusion of nitroprusside, which by 1973 had become our standard therapy for shock caused by heart failure. Joe immediately had a favorable response with improved circulation, better urine output and gradual relief of his pulmonary congestion. But there was a problem. Every time we tried to wean him off the nitroprusside infusion, his condition dramatically worsened.

He began walking around the ward dragging his IV pole with the nitroprusside dripping into his vein. After a week of continuous infusion of nitroprusside, his blood levels of the toxic by-product of nitroprusside, thiocyanate, began to rise and it was clear that we had to find an alternative approach to therapy. In the absence of an established treatment we administered isosorbide dinitrate by mouth and nitroglycerin ointment on the skin, each given four times a day on a staggered schedule. If we had known about the value of adding hydralazine to the nitrate we would have done so. But we didn't learn about hydralazine until four years later.

Nonetheless, the nitrate therapy seemed to have a favorable effect. Over the next few days we gradually tapered his nitroprusside infusion until it had been discontinued. The oral and skin nitrates were maintained, and he was subsequently discharged and instructed to take both treatments around the clock at 4-hour intervals—a dose of isosorbide dinitrate, followed two hours later by nitroglycerin ointment, then followed two hours later with another isosorbide dinitrate tablet.

The burden of this every two hour treatment did not discourage Joe or his wife. An alarm clock helped him maintain the treatment throughout the night. I saw him in clinic every few weeks. He was maintaining an active lifestyle and was free of symptoms.

On one of his visits, however, a new medical resident who was working with me became skeptical that Joe's nitrate therapy was having any effect. The literature was still ambiguous as to whether nitrates taken either by mouth or on the skin exerted any effect. I was willing to test the hypothesis.

Without Mr. or Mrs. Abbey's knowledge, I substituted a placebo tablet for the isosorbide dinitrate and allowed him to continue using the ointment. In those days, informed consent for administering a placebo was not required. Joe went home with a new bottle of medication and instructions to return in two weeks to be re-evaluated. Five days later I received a hysterical call from Mrs. Abbey. Joe had gradually been getting worse since he had seen me in clinic and was now back in his full-blown heart failure state—unable to breathe, weak, and semiconscious. He was rushed to the hospital where we reinstituted his oral isosorbide dinitrate. He promptly recovered and returned to his previous active lifestyle. I felt remorse for putting Joe and his wife through this ordeal. I told them what I had done and they were remarkably forgiving.

This single-blind study (in which I knew but the patient didn't) had certainly proved to my satisfaction that the oral nitrate was effective and that it was, perhaps along with the ointment, maintaining improved left ventricular function in this patient. I suspected Sam Farber would have responded the same way as Joe.

Now we had evidence that the combination of isosorbide dinitrate and hydralazine was even better. It could replicate the effect of nitroprusside. So we were ready to embark on a trial with a combination of isosorbide dinitrate and hydralazine as a vasodilator regimen hoping that it would produce a sustained hemodynamic effect favorably influencing the long-term outcome in patients with heart failure.

As noted earlier, we were also interested in exploring drugs that might interfere with the mechanisms of artery constriction. Our hormone studies had identified three possible contributors to artery constriction: norepinephrine, renin and vasopressin. In the late 1970s, efforts to develop oral drugs to inhibit renin and vasopressin were in their infancy—certainly not ready for a clinical trial in heart failure. There was, however, considerable clinical experience in hypertension with drugs that block the vasoconstrictor activity of norepinephrine. We and others had studied prazosin, called an alpha blocker because it inhibits the constrictor action of norepinephrine on the wall of arteries and veins. Prazosin therapy would provide a way to compare the effectiveness of a drug combination that dilates the blood vessels with a single drug that interferes with the constriction induced by the sympathetic nervous system. We wanted to conduct a clinical trial to test these two oral regimens against a placebo in patients receiving standard background therapy for heart failure.

A new V.A. trial

We turned again to the V.A. Cooperative Studies program because now we had not only an important long-term question to answer, but we had a group of investigators who had already worked together on the no-name nitroprusside study and were prepared to embark on a trial in chronic heart failure. No such trials in heart failure had yet been conducted. No new therapy had been developed in a generation. Standard treatment was a diuretic to relieve the body of excess fluid and digoxin, an old drug derived from the foxglove plant, *digitalis purpurea,* that had been studied by my pharmacologist uncle Harry Gold.

But we were talking here about a long-term study—not the 90-day outcome that we had focused on in the nitroprusside trial, but a long-term outcome study of perhaps four or five years. Such an undertaking would be expensive. We needed a protocol. We had to have drugs man-ufactured. We needed investigator meetings.

We needed an acronym.

Yes, we wanted a study to show if chronic therapy with a drug that was not designed to *stimulate the heart* but rather to *relax the blood vessels* could prolong life in patients with heart failure. if it worked, we also wanted to understand why it was effective.

I was fixated on function of the left ventricle, the relationship be-tween filling pressure and cardiac output—the old Frank-Starling curve. Our drugs were effective in improving function—we thought we were testing the long-term benefit of improving left ventricular function.

I vowed we would not only monitor morbidity and mortality—the outcomes to show whether our treatment was effective—but also se-quentially monitor the function of the left ventricle so that we could try to relate the functional improvement to the outcome benefit.

At that time, we could not appreciate that this was to be the first of a clinical trial model that has dominated cardiovascular clinical research over the past 30 years.

I was optimistic and excited. We had the opportunity to document effectiveness of the first new drug for heart failure in the modern era. I dreamed of treating Sam Farber with this new drug. In my dream, I instructed an appreciative Sam and Naomi about how to take the drug.

CHAPTER VIII
Vasodilator-Heart Failure Trial (V-HeFT)

Planning a long-term clinical trial is a complicated venture. First of all trials are expensive, so you need funding to embark on the process. In 1979, I decided to once again approach the V.A. Cooperative Studies office for support of a study in chronic heart failure. We needed a hypothesis that would be attractive to the review committee of clinicians and scientists. We needed collaborating investigators at other V.A. Hospitals willing to participate in the study. Since our goal was to test drugs, we needed a source of the medication, hopefully along with some pharmaceutical company support. And most importantly, we needed a protocol for patient management that all participants could agree to follow.

The hypothesis was simple and very attractive. Heart failure was (and still is) an increasingly common condition resulting in frequent hospitalizations within the Veterans Administration health care system. Morbidity and mortality from heart failure was very high and management was remarkably unsatisfactory. Diuretics were available to relieve patients of the congestion and swelling which impaired the quality of their lives. Digitalis, on old drug purified from the foxglove plant, was the only other agent frequently used to treat patients, but its effectiveness was modest at best and side effects (sudden death from a rhythm disturbance was the most dramatic) led to questions about whether it should be routinely employed.

Years later, the NIH would fund a large study to determine if digoxin, the most widely used form of digitalis, could save lives. It was a "large, simple trial" in which the only thing monitored was death. The results did not really resolve the controversy. Overall, there was no benefit of digoxin. There might have been a slight decrease in deaths due to heart failure, but this slight benefit appeared to be counterbalanced by a slight increase in "sudden death". The investigators' proposed that the excess sudden deaths might be due to a heart rhythm abnormality induced by the digoxin.

The drug's use in practice had remained arbitrary. There were no other drugs available for the condition, and the disease appeared to be progressive. Thus the concept of a new therapeutic agent to be employed to alter the progressive, downhill course of congestive heart failure was attractive to the V.A, as it would have been to any health care organization.

An acronym

Naturally, we needed an acronym. A study identified by a number would hardly be effective in gaining world-wide attention. We needed a title that was easy to pronounce, but I was intolerant to study names that were manipulated into a word that tried to make a statement. The NIH, for instance, started a trial in individuals they thought were at high risk for a heart attack. They decided to call it the "Multiple Risk Factor Intervention Trial", perhaps because the initials of the words were MRFIT. It was commonly referred to as "Mister Fit", although purists insisted on pronouncing it "Murfit".

After considering a number of letter combinations that could be created from potential titles of the study, I settled on "Vasodilator Heart Failure Trial" or V-HeFT. I insisted, for purity, to keep the "e" in lower case, since it was derived from the "e" in heart, not from the first letter of a word.

Pharmaceutical company support

The two vasodilator drugs (isosorbide dinitrate and hydralazine) that we had combined to produce the favorable effect on heart function described earlier were generic agents available by prescription. The most commonly used forms of these drugs were Isordil, manufactured by Ives Laboratories, and Apresoline, manufactured by Ciba Pharmaceuticals. The other vasodilator drug we wanted to test was prazosin, manufactured as Minipres by Pfizer.

I approached management of these pharmaceutical companies to see if they would support the project by providing medication, as well as some financial aid. All three companies agreed to participate. I suspect their willingness to collaborate was based more on the scientific challenge than the potential for profit. None of them saw much of a market for their drug in this endeavor, and as far as Isordil and Apresoline were concerned, the generic nature of these products meant that the price was low and any competing manufacturer could produce the drug.

I approached my V.A. colleagues who participated in Study 19, the no-name nitroprusside trial. All but two sites enthusiastically agreed to continue our collaboration. I identified two additional V.A. Hospitals where my recent trainees had taken staff positions. They were delighted to join us. Again we had 11 centers ready to recruit patients. I brought together a planning group, composed of a few of these investigators and a biostatistician, assigned by the V.A. Cooperative Studies office, to work with us on protocol development.

Trial design

As previously noted, the biostatistician's role in designing a clinical trial is a critical one. Trials test a hypothesis, and the statistical power to confirm the hypothesis is related to the trial design and the outcomes being measured. In statistical terms, and quite paradoxically, the goal is to reject the null or "no effect" hypothesis. Since our aim was to reduce mortality with drug therapy in heart failure, our statistical goal was to reject the null hypothesis that the mortality in the patients randomly assigned to take the experimental treatment was the same as the mortality in the control arm that received a dummy drug (placebo). That means that the number of deaths in the treatment arm needed to be so much lower than the number of deaths in the control arm that the likelihood of that happening by chance was less than 1 in 20.

That statistical power, or a P value <0.05, is the traditional standard of proof. This doesn't mean that a P value of less than .05 (1 in 20) means that the differences could not have occurred by chance alone, but that the likelihood of that occurrence is so low that scientists have agreed it is adequate to reject the null hypothesis.

What makes a P<0.05 so magical? Nothing, really, except tradition. Isn't a 9 in 10 chance (P=0.1) adequate evidence for a favorable effect? It may be, but biostatisticians, regulatory bodies and most scientists won't accept it. And this issue would ultimately become very important.

Existing data were inadequate to properly calculate the number of patients needed in the trial. No previous trials had been carried out in patients with heart failure, so although we knew the mortality rate would be high, we did not know exactly how high. Furthermore, we had no experience with the planned drug therapies, and consequently didn't know what magnitude of benefit to expect. These were the early days of clinical trials. Very few had been carried out in advanced cardiovascular disease. I insisted to the biostatistician that we couldn't use traditional approaches to calculate the power and devise the number of patients required to address the hypothesis. Instead, I estimated the number of patients that I thought the 11 centers could recruit and asked the statistician to calculate the power we could achieve with that number of patients based on our prediction of mortality rate. It was an unusual approach which, fortunately, was accepted by the V.A. Cooperative Studies review committee.

We designed the study with three treatment arms. All patients would be given standard therapy with diuretics and digoxin. The control group would receive a placebo, one treatment group would receive prazosin— the alpha adrenergic blocker manufactured by Pfizer—and the other treatment group would receive a combination of hydralazine manufactured by Ciba, and isosorbide dinitrate manufactured by Ives Laboratories.

It was unusual at that time and rarer since to get pharmaceutical companies to work together. Since the study needed to be double-blind-ed (neither the patient nor the health care personnel could know which treatment the patients were taking), I had to negotiate with the three companies to produce appropriate medication. We finally decided that the hydralazine and the prazosin could each be placed into a capsule (although they were marketed in a tablet form) that would look identi-cal. It would also be easy to provide a placebo capsule that would con-tain a powdery milk substance with no therapeutic effect. The isosor-bide dinitrate came in a tablet formulation. Ives Laboratories offered to provide a matching placebo. Therefore, the design of the study was quite practical.

The control group would receive a placebo capsule and a placebo tablet four times daily. This group would represent the standard therapy of the day with digoxin and diuretic. The two treatment groups would also receive a capsule and a tablet four times daily. But in one group the capsule would be prazosin and the tablet would be placebo, and in the other group the capsule would be hydralazine and the tablet would be isosorbide dinitrate.

A further complication was that we wanted to start everyone on a low dose, in case of side effects, and then go up to the target dose. Therefore, the experimental drugs were provided as pills or capsules containing half the drug dose we wanted to give. This meant our target dose would re-quire *two* tablets and *two* capsules four times daily, or 16 medication dos-es a day. Formulating these products, packaging them with appropriate numerical labels and developing a randomization scheme and appropri-ate code numbers were processes well established in clinical trials.

With the biostatistician, we decided to aim for a study of 720 pa-tients. Since there was no prior experience with outcomes in patients with heart failure treated with the standard digoxin-diuretic medication, we felt we should randomize more patients to the placebo arm than to ei-ther treatment arm. This would allow us to have a more reliable estimate of outcome in patients on standard therapy for heart failure. We devised a randomization schema that was based on sets of seven patients in each center, with three of the set randomized to placebo and two to each of the treatments. Therefore, we knew that after every seven patients randomized at each center, 3 would have received placebo and two would have received each of the other drug treatments. Of course, none of our trial staff would know which patients received which treatment.

Based on our estimate from crude clinical records of a 20% annual mortality in the placebo group, this was calculated to provide us with 84% power to detect a 33% reduction in mortality (20% to 13.4% annual mortality). Furthermore, this distribution of treatments would give us maximum power if we chose to merge the two treatment groups (after all, they were both vasodilator regimens and that is what we thought we were studying) and compare the merged treatment group with the placebo group.

The power concept is a rather arcane biostatistical principle. What the estimates suggested is that if we were mostly correct in our prediction of control group mortality, we should be able to detect the kind of benefit we were seeking.

By current standards, the study was under-powered and should have been much larger. A 90% power calculation is usually required these days, thus reducing the risk of what is called a beta error: failing to identify a difference even though the difference exists. And seeking a 33% reduction in mortality would be viewed these days as wildly optimistic. But we were limited by logistics and budget to 11 centers and their local restraints on finding and randomizing suitable patients.

The decision about who to include in the trial was critical. Doctors may know how to diagnose congestive heart failure, but a clinical trial requires precise criteria for patient entrance. Since the hallmark of heart failure is fatigue and shortness of breath on exertion, these were the symptom-based entrance criteria. Patients with heart failure generally have an enlarged heart divulged by chest x-ray. X-ray evidence of cardiac enlargement was therefore an additional entrance criterion.

We wanted to be more precise. There was growing recognition that weakness of the heart's contraction is a critical contributor to heart failure and resulting morbidity and mortality. Therefore, we felt it would be important to assess what was called the "left ventricular ejection fraction" as an entrance criterion. If you measure the amount of blood in the left ventricle before the next beat of the heart, *ejection fraction* is the percentage of that blood which is pumped out with that next beat. The normal left ventricle may contain a volume of 150 ml, or about five ounces of blood at the end of the filling phase of the cardiac cycle (diastole). It may eject 100 ml. with each beat. So the ejection fraction (EF) would be 100/150, or 67%.

The conventional wisdom was that ejection fraction, or EF, was the best way to assess heart function. The weaker its contraction, the smaller the fraction of its contained blood would be ejected with each beat. We have since learned, as discussed later, that it is more complicated than that.

The most quantitative method for measuring ejection fraction, and one not prone to observer bias, is a radionuclide method in which an isotope tracer is injected into the circulating blood to label the blood cells, and then a nuclear detector is placed over the heart to assess the change in counts during each contraction of the left ventricle. This is generally an expensive procedure because of the requirements of complex equipment, a highly-trained technician, and a nuclear tracer. Since all the participating V.A. Hospitals had available to them a nuclear laboratory capable of carrying out these studies, this appeared to be a valuable entrance criterion. We chose an ejection fraction of less than 45% as an entrance criterion to avoid including "normals", those with values of 50% or higher. We decided to enter patients who met either the chest X-ray criterion of an enlarged heart shadow or the ejection fraction criterion, since we knew there would be some who would not meet both criteria. This decision was remarkably fortunate. We have come to realize that many patients with heart failure (up to half in some studies) do not have a reduced left ventricular ejection fraction but may have an enlarged heart shadow on X-ray (heart failure with preserved ejection fraction.) To facilitate conversations about heart failure with a preserved ejection fraction, this has come to be called HFpEF, pronounced "Hefpef,"

We now suspect that these latter patients—often elderly and more commonly women—have symptoms of heart failure because of a stiff left ventricle that does not fill easily rather than a left ventricle that does not empty properly. The enlarged cardiac silhouette on X-ray in these patients represents enlargement of the right ventricle and atria, which are distended, not the left ventricle which is stiff. Symptoms come primarily from the high filling pressure in the left ventricle, which is not accompanied by a large volume (Figure VIII-1). Since the left ventricle is not dilated, and its stroke volume is maintained by a high filling pressure, the ejection fraction remains normal.

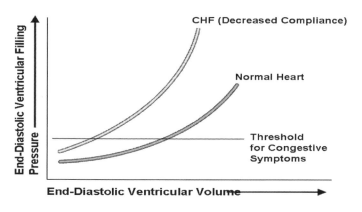

Figure VIII-1

The compliance or distensibility of the left ventricle is defined by the pressure-volume relationship. If the left ventricle stiffens, as it usually does during aging, a smaller increase in volume will result in a greater rise in pressure. When that pressure exceeds a certain threshold level, symptoms of lung congestion will occur. Therefore, heart failure can occur without an enlarged left ventricle.

This finding therefore represents an exception to our prior hypothesis that a high filling pressure in the left ventricle is associated with a high volume. Ejection fraction may be normal in such situations, but the Frank-Starling relationship (Figure III-3) is abnormal. Ejection fraction (EF), therefore, is not always a guide to the Frank-Starling curve. By including both cardiac enlargement and ejection fraction as eligibility criteria, we were able to recruit both kinds of heart failure—that which is currently identified as low EF, and that which is identified as normal or preserved EF.

The issue of gender

Patient selection required another critical decision. I was an advocate for homogeneous populations in studies. Other clinical trialists have embarked on large-scale trials in widely diverse populations in hopes of establishing a treatment that could be applicable to the whole population. I was concerned about heterogeneity of response and wanted to avoid diversity unless we could be certain of adequate numbers in each subgroup.

In the 1970s, V.A. Hospitals predominantly had male patients. Females served in the military in various capacities and women were admitted with heart failure. However, I recognized that the number of women would be so small that it would be impossible to analyze them separately and it would be inappropriate to assume their response to therapy was identical to that of men. I made the decision to confine the patient population to males. In light of subsequent events and current emphasis on subgroups, it was the right decision, although today it probably would be viewed as prejudiced against women.

There's more to life than death

Another decision had greater implications. Although our primary endpoint for the trial was to be mortality, it was clear to me that other manifestations of the disease process were of considerable importance to patients. Exercise intolerance is a primary manifestation of heart failure, and it is often the symptom most troublesome to patients. Since our goal of therapy was not only to prolong life but also to make people feel better, I felt that we should include in the protocol some objective measure of exercise tolerance before and after treatment was initiated. The most precise way to assess exercise tolerance is to measure the maximum amount of work a patient can do by assessing his oxygen consumption at the peak of his exercise capacity. This is rather cumbersome methodology, requiring the patient to exercise with a tube in his mouth and his nose clamped off. Thus all the air entering the lungs passes through the tube in the mouth and all the exhaled air passes through the tube and into a sensor which continuously monitors oxygen and carbon dioxide in the air. This technique requires instrumentation that all the centers agreed to accept as part of the protocol. An abnormally low peak exercise oxygen consumption—that is, reduced exercise capacity—therefore became another entrance criterion for participating in the study. Finally, then, we embarked on the largest scale study ever carried out using exercise gas exchange to calculate oxygen consumption during exercise.

We formed an Executive Steering Committee which included representatives from each of the three drug companies along with a few senior lead investigators who oversaw the conduct of the trial. It was a remarkable example of collegial spirit, largely because we were breaking new ground with a disease that had not yet been subjected to careful study, and we were using drugs that none of the manufacturers had any interest in developing for heart failure. The pharma companies were doing it in the spirit of creative research and we investigators were doing it for the joy of discovery, a contribution to medical knowledge and management, and the possibility of important publications.

Another feature of V-HeFT was made possible because it was carried out exclusively in Veterans Administration hospitals. The V.A., of course, is a socialized health care system. The patients did not pay for their care, insurance companies were not involved, and the doctors were salaried. The cost of procedures was borne by the hospital, and the V.A. Cooperative Studies were an integral part of the hospital's healthcare responsibility.

I made the decision at the outset that we could not do a mortality trial in heart failure without collecting a host of other data to test the severity of the disease and its response to therapy. Rather than carry out these mechanistic substudies in a small fraction of the overall study population, as is common practice today, I insisted that we should do such studies in the entire population in order to more accurately track the progression of the disease and the effectiveness of therapy. This made the protocol far more burdensome, but it provided us with a wealth of data that ultimately served as the foundation for much of what we now know about heart failure. Therefore, all patients in V-HeFT underwent sequential exercise testing, all patients underwent sequential measurements of ejection fraction over time, most patients had ultrasound imaging of their hearts (echocardiography), and most had sequential monitoring of their electrocardiograms for 24 hours (Holter monitoring).

These all would have been exorbitantly expensive tests if performed in private institutions—or in any healthcare environment today—but in the 1980s we pulled it off, thanks to the socialized V.A. system.

Esprits de corps

As we put the final touches on the protocol, we gathered the potential investigators to discuss details. The 11 principal investigators from 11 V.A. Hospitals all came to Minneapolis along with the nurse that each had appointed as its local study coordinator. A physician at each center served as Principal Investigator with responsibility for patient care and quality control. But the day-to-day conduct of such a study is critically dependent on the coordinators, who must communicate regularly with the patients, see them when they come to be evaluated, and organize the collection of data. These individuals are usually nurses who have decided to become fulltime research coordinators funded by the study budget. The success of the study in an individual institution is usually dependent on the dedication and skill of these nurses. Their presence at our initial meeting was a critical factor in the study's success.

It has always been my philosophy that strong centralized management of a trial is mandatory in order to guarantee the quality of the data collected. Therefore, another feature critical to the success of V-HeFT was the management skill of Susan Ziesche, the nurse who had begun to work with me on Study 19 several years earlier. Susan became the glue that held V-HeFT together. Her organizational skill and her close relationship to all the nurses in the 11 participating centers were critical to management decisions in the individual centers and to the quality of the data collected.

At that first meeting, it became clear that this group, most of whom knew each other from the previous study, was going to be a cohesive study group. Our dinner gatherings (now held at a local restaurant because of eviction from our house) helped to weld the group together.

Despite the camaraderie of the group and the dedication to a successful trial, recruitment lagged. As we've come to learn, recruitment of patients into clinical trials always goes more slowly than planned. There are many reasons for this. The protocol's entrance criteria exclude many patients who might otherwise be eligible. Patients may have disease characteristics that make them ineligible. They may be receiving drug therapy that excludes them. They may have coexistent diseases which limit their participation. Or they may not agree to participate.

There is also the problem of finding patients. These individuals are often under care of private physicians or hospital physicians and may not be identified by the study team. Even if one were to find them, some of them may have primary care physicians who do not want them to participate in the trial. So one of the major activities of the study's nursing personnel was to form a good working relationship with physicians around the hospital or in the clinic to help them identify eligible patients and refer them for participation.

Eventually, the V.A. Cooperative Studies office expressed concern about the expense of the study and the relatively small number of patients recruited for participation. It began calculating a figure representing the cost per patient based on the overall budget and the number of patients actually recruited and randomized into the trial. These figures never made us look good in comparison to other clinical trials, but the bureaucrats failed to recognize the complexity of the study, the burden on our personnel in carrying out the required studies, and the importance of the disease we were investigating. It was nonetheless clear that the motivation of the investigators and their study coordinators was a critical factor. After each investigator meeting a bump in recruitment was always noted, implying that we needed to get their attention in order to actively recruit patients. Susan was the key to this aggressive motivational effort and her frequent phone calls with each coordinator began to pay dividends.

One of the strategies was "guilt and shame". We began publishing a regular newsletter which served as a vehicle to keep the V-HeFT investigators up-to-date on protocol amendments and compliance issues. But on a regular basis the newsletter also reported the performance of individual centers. Nothing was more embarrassing for a center than to discover its recruitment was below that of everyone else. Thus, with a combination of regular phone calls, motivational speeches and embarrassing standings, the study's recruitment picked up.

The problems of unblinding and compliance

Getting patients into a trial is one thing, but keeping them actively participating for its entire duration, which in V-HeFT extended to five years, was quite another challenge. Coordinators had to deal with a host of unexpected issues. One patient, a 53-year old business man from Nashville, decided to take his medications to a local laboratory for analysis. When he reported back to the clinic that he had learned he was taking prazosin, it created a problem because his participation was no longer blinded. The only solution was to "censor" his data and terminate him from the study. Censoring means that follow-up ceases at the time of the event, which in this case was the unblinding of the patient.

A more conventional unblinding event occurred in Chicago. A 61-year-old man developed some joint pains that his local physician felt might be lupus, a serious potential complication of hydralazine therapy, especially with high doses. The possibility of this complication was carefully described in the study consent form, even though we had never seen a case of lupus with the modest doses of hydralazine being used in V-HeFT. Our usual approach with such events was to suggest that the study drug be discontinued to see if the symptoms disappeared. Unblinding should not be necessary and the patient can continue in the trial even if he stops taking the drug. Indeed, the randomization process places the patient in a treatment group forever, whether he continues on the treatment or not.

In this case, the patient's physician would not accept this advice. He demanded to know what drug his patient was receiving. That information is always available in a sealed envelope for situations where the identity of the drug becomes critical for management, or in instances where it is demanded by health care providers. We opened the envelope and he was on placebo. He was censored at that point.

One of the features of a drug trial is the monitoring of compliance with the therapy. Patients are instructed to bring back their pill bottles at each visit. They usually appear in the clinic carrying a paper bag that contains the pill bottles dispensed at the last visit. The idea, of course, is for the coordinator to count the pills, which have been carefully counted when dispensed so that there would be about five day's supply left when the patient returned. Of course, the patient could discard untaken pills to place their compliance in a favorable light, but they rarely appear to do that. They may come in with a month's supply left and try to claim that they "never miss a dose". Careful questioning usually reveals the compliance problem and the nurses spend considerable time helping to improve adherence. Such experience with patients who should be motivated to comply because of their agreement to participate helps to better understand therapeutic failures in regular medical practice. Patients simply cannot remember to take their pills. We have all had the experience of being prescribed a drug—for instance, a 7-day supply of an antibiotic—only to find that at the end of seven days there are still a number of capsules left in the bottle. The truth comes out in a controlled clinical trial.

The monitoring board

All outcome trials in sick patients require oversight from a Data Safety and Monitoring Board (DSMB). This board is appointed to protect the patients who have agreed to participate in the study. They are patient advocates even though the patients never get to meet them. Their goal is to monitor progression of the study data and to oversee complications, side effects, and mortality rates to assure that the patients are not being adversely affected by their participation. This involves monitoring sequentially any difference in outcome between the control arm and the treatment arms that might mandate early termination of the trial or modification of the protocol.

I appointed to the DSMB two cardiologists, one pharmacologist who was familiar with the drugs we were using, and one biostatistician whose role was to oversee the statistical calculations. All data were collected in a coordinating center operated by the V.A. in West Haven, Connecticut, and the biostatistician assigned by the V.A. to the study served as the keeper of all the data. As the Study Chairman, I was blinded to the treatment arms, which in this case were identified as Treatment A, Treatment B, and Treatment C. The DSMB had the right to unblind itself at any time it was felt that unblinding would enhance its ability to provide proper oversight.

Patients are recruited to enter a clinical trial over a period of time. In V-HeFT it took us more than three years to accumulate what we thought was an adequate sample size, 640 patients rather than the 720 patients we had initially projected. In V.A. trials at the time, all the data were sent from the individual clinical centers (where the standardized forms were completed by the study coordinators) to the V.A. data support center, where the data were entered into a computer for analysis. These data were then provided in a coded form to the Data Safety and Monitoring Board (DSMB), which is empowered to track the adverse events in the three treatment groups. These outcome data were provided with great secrecy to the DSMB and were not viewed by anyone involved in conducting the trial. The secrecy of this process is elaborately maintained by unique coding maneuvers, private mailings, and destruction of all printed material as soon as each meeting of the DSMB has ended.

As study chairman I was not privy to the unblinded data. I knew the overall experience in the study but not the outcomes in the three treatment groups. These data were made available to the members of the DSMB, with whom I met at each of their gatherings to provide an update on the conduct of the trial and any problems encountered. So I did become aware of some of their complex deliberations.

The initial plan was to monitor the outcome in the three treatment arms independently. But we anticipated that the two drug treatment arms, which were designed to relax the blood vessels and reduce the burden on the heart, would exhibit a similar benefit and thus the two arms might be merged in analysis to compare with the results in the placebo arm, which represented standard heart failure therapy at that time.

Why do patients die?

Although the statistical goal was to compare all-cause mortality in the three treatment arms of V-HeFT, it was apparent that we needed to analyze mechanism of death. As part of the responsibility of the principal investigators at each center, a death form was completed for each patient who died during the course of the trial. That form required the investigator to check off the apparent cause of the patient's death. If the patient were observed to die suddenly carrying out normal life activities, the box could be checked for sudden death. If the patient was found dead but not observed during his terminal episode, we encouraged staff members to use their best judgment in identifying it as a sudden unobserved death or as some other mechanism. If the patient had been hospitalized and was clearly exhibiting signs of worsening heart failure before he died, the death was classified as pump failure or heart failure death. Obviously, many episodes were not easily classifiable and the principal investigator was given the option of using his or her best judgment. It was usually the study coordinator, not the doctor, who knew most about the patient's final episode.

I was dissatisfied with this process because there was no overall quality control. As part of the instructions for monitoring patients at the individual centers, I asked that a narrative be provided to detail the prior events surrounding the terminal episode so that an independent judgment could be made. Mode of death could be important, because a sudden death, presumably from an electrical failure of the heart's rhythm, might be preventable with other therapy. But a pump failure death would suggest that our treatment had failed to support heart function in that patient. In recent years, it has become standard practice to implant a cardiac defibrillator in patients with heart failure to counteract death from a rhythm disturbance.

The process of assigning mechanism of death is now referred to as an event adjudication committee. This committee is usually made up of investigators in the trial, but sometimes of outside individuals. Committee members are provided data much as we were collecting in V-HeFT and asked to adjudicate the mechanism of death or, if hospitalizations were to be adjudicated, the cause of the hospitalization. It is critical that the committee be unaware of the treatment assignment of the patients. These event committees often are asked to review hundreds of events that need adjudication. The committee members then vote on each event to reach a consensus that becomes the final results. The process is laborious but democratic.

In the late 1980s, the process of adjudication and the structure of such event committees had not been established. Therefore, I undertook a simplified version of this process. All the supporting data relating to a terminal event in an individual patient were provided to me. Susan Ziesche and I then sat down and reviewed each of the cases in detail and reached a conclusion as to whether the death could be attributed to a sudden event, a progressive pump failure event, a sudden event associated with premonitory worsening of symptoms, some other cardiovascular event such as stroke or aneurysm or procedural complication, or a death related to a non-cardiovascular cause such as cancer.

The most dramatic example of this latter category was a 54-year-old man, who apparently was feeling quite well on his therapy in V-HeFT and was involved in an extra-marital relationship. His wife found him in bed with his lover and shot him. It was clearly a sudden death, but we decided that it was non-cardiovascular. Nonetheless, as in all clinical trials, the death was counted in the treatment arm to which he was randomized. Even though he was clearly quite functional, his death—like all deaths in an all-cause mortality trail—could influence our interpretation of the effectiveness of the treatment to which he was assigned. This is a potential weakness of all mortality trials, but fortunately, from a statistical point-of-view, such events are overwhelmed in trials like V-HeFT with deaths from a cardiac cause.

But separation of cardiac causes from non-cardiac causes can be more difficult than in the philanderer described above. Did the auto accident result from a heart rhythm disturbance while at the wheel, or was it an unrelated driver error? Would the pneumonia have killed this patient if he did not have severe heart disease?

End-point analysis

Deaths began to accumulate early in the trial. Indeed, within the first year it became apparent to the DSMB that the mortality rate in two of the three arms was approaching our estimated annual rate of 20 percent. In the third arm, however, the mortality rate appeared to be lower. That difference continued to expand as the trial went on and the DSMB regularly met at 6-month intervals. The Board recognized the need to be certain that the lower mortality rate was not occurring in the placebo arm, because if it were, the study might need to be terminated early because of an adverse trend with the experimental treatments.

It wasn't.

Although I was not made aware of this issue, the group treated with isosorbide dinitrate and hydralazine was exhibiting a lower mortality rate than the other two arms. The other vasodilator arm—prazosin— was tracking precisely with the placebo arm. The DSMB had no intention to merge the treatment arms for analysis. The two vasodilator arms were not responding similarly.

When V-HeFT was completed and the data analyzed, the investigators and the DSMB concluded that the isosorbide dinitrate/hydralazine arm exhibited a lower mortality than the placebo arm. The P value for this difference we calculated as $P = 0.046$, meaning that there was a less than 5% chance (1 in 20) that this difference in outcome could have occurred by chance. When we subsequently published the manuscript, we identified the P value as less than 0.05 and concluded that the isosorbide dinitrate/hydralazine combination had exerted a significantly favorable effect on life expectancy in patients with heart failure (Figure VIII-2).

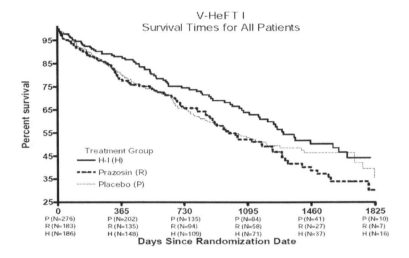

Figure VIII-2

Survival times in the three treatment groups in V-HeFT. The number of patients (N) included at each time point is shown below the graph. Survival was improved with isosorbide dinitrate-hydralazine treatment (H-I) compared to prazosin or placebo. The p-value for the benefit of H-I was 0.046.

Although the statistical significance of the mortality benefit could be interpreted as "borderline" because the p-value just made the significance threshold, the magnitude of the life-saving effect of the drug combination was quite striking. The small sample size is responsible for that discrepancy. By one year after randomization, nearly 20% of the placebo patients had died compared to 12% of the isosorbide dinitrate-hydralazine patients, a 40% reduction in mortality. That means that if you were to treat 100 patients with heart failure, eight would have been kept alive who would otherwise have died. At two and three years, the number saved increased to 9 and 10. These results provide a powerful example of the difference between absolute and relative risk reduction in clinical trials.

The media often hype a new observation that claims to demonstrate a profound reduction in mortality, for instance a 50% decrease in some morbid event. When one examines the data, however, one finds that it may be a decrease from a 0.2% risk to a 0.1% risk. The absolute risk reduction is therefore preciously small, even though the relative risk reduction appears large. In V-HeFT the relative and absolute risk reduction were both substantial.

The paradox of heart function

The dramatic results from V-HeFT raised many fascinating questions. It was the first time it had been demonstrated that the course of heart failure could be altered by therapy. What was the mechanism that mediated this benefit? If it was vasodilation by relaxing the arteries, why didn't prazosin also exert a favorable effect? Our carefully planned studies of left ventricular function gave us the exciting clue.

In patients given ISDN and hydralazine, we observed a consistent increase in ejection fraction; that is, the function of the heart appeared to improve, and the improved function was maintained over time. In the groups given prazosin or placebo, the ejection fraction progressively declined. Therefore, our drug combination had a remarkable and apparently unique effect on the heart that was not shared by another vasodilator.

To study the heart function, we had employed a nuclear technique that measured the fraction of blood ejected with each beat of the left ventricle, the "ejection fraction". That measurement was (and in many clinics still is) viewed as the best measure of the function of the heart. Since ejection fraction rose in the ISDN/HYD treated group, we immediately assumed that the drug combination, by reducing impedance, had allowed better emptying of the heart. But if so, why didn't prazosin, a known vasodilator, do the same thing? It wasn't that prazosin was a weaker vasodilator. In fact, blood pressure was reduced in the prazosin group, a manifestation of its vasodilator effect, whereas it did not significantly decline in the ISDN/HYD group.

The solution to this paradox came to me in the shower one morning. The fraction of blood ejected with each beat is very dependent on the volume in the left ventricle at the time of its contraction. For the same volume, a greater ejection fraction would mean a more forceful contraction and a higher stroke volume or cardiac output. Under these circumstances, the ejection fraction is a measure of function. But what if the volume in the chamber before contraction has increased, as it would have with structural remodeling and chamber enlargement? (Figure VIII-3).

To eject the same stroke volume from a larger volume would now require a lower ejection fraction. If the end-diastolic volume is now 300 ml. rather than 150 ml, a normal stroke volume of 100 ml. would appear to maintain adequate blood flow—but now with an ejection fraction of 100/300, or 33%, rather than 67%.

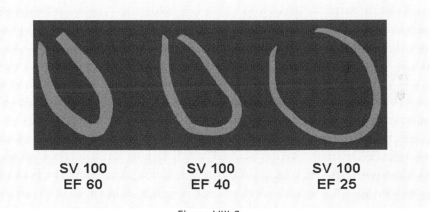

SV 100   SV 100   SV 100
EF 60   EF 40   EF 25

Figure VIII-3

Diagram of the left ventricle. The normal-sized chamber (left) in order to eject a stroke volume of 100 ml. might have an ejection fraction of 60%. As the chamber enlarges because of remodeling (center and right) 100 ml. can be ejected with a much lower ejection fraction. A low ejection fraction, therefore, is a consequence of an enlarging chamber, not necessarily impaired pumping function of the heart.

Under these circumstances, therefore, a fall in EF is a manifestation of structural remodeling of the heart, not of impaired function. And an increase in EF, as we had observed with ISDN/HYD in V-HeFT, could signify regression of remodeling, not a unique effect on function. Was the ISDN-hydralazine combination exerting a favorable structural effect on the heart?

We turned back to a dog model of heart muscle damage that will be described in the next chapter. We performed a new series of experiments in which we damaged the dog's left ventricle and then began treatment with different drugs. When we gave ISDN, progressive enlargement of the heart was blocked. But when we gave an alpha blocker, like prazosin, there was no inhibition of the remodeling effect. Our clinical studies had led us to the animal laboratory for confirmation.

It was a reversal of the currently popular concept of "Translational Research", which suggests that discoveries are made in the laboratory and then applied in the clinic. We did it the other way around.

We had many questions to pursue after analyzing the results of V-HeFT, but the first priority was to present and publish our findings. That occurred in a high-profile presentation at the annual meeting of the American Heart Association in 1985, and in a prominent report in the *New England Journal of Medicine* in 1986. The first new therapy for heart failure in a generation had emerged as life-saving. This would become the new standard treatment, we thought, because the drugs were readily available by prescription and were inexpensive.

Our marketing disadvantage

But we underestimated the complexity of introducing a new therapy into clinical practice. Doctors are remarkably set in their ways. They don't hear or read about a new therapy and immediately start using it. Pharmaceutical companies addressed this inertia problem in multiple ways. They hire thousands of sales people who visit doctors to convince them of the value of a new drug. They organize and sponsor lectures by thought leaders, often accompanied by lunch or dinner, to promote their company-sponsored studies. They send out glossy mailings with accompanying trinkets. In more recent years, they discovered that the most effective marketing may be directly to the patient. It is hard to watch TV these days without being engulfed by drug company promotion for a therapy that "you should ask your doctor about".

We were at a hopeless disadvantage. We had no corporate sponsor for our therapy, no marketing budget, and in fact no marketing. All we had was a report in the *New England Journal of Medicine* and accompanying media coverage, which was over in two days and forgotten soon after.

Physicians are free to prescribe approved drugs they think are effective, even in medical conditions for which the drugs are not approved. But drugs cannot be labeled or promoted for a use which has not been approved by the Food and Drug Administration. Approval, therefore, was critical if we were to achieve wider use of this life-saving therapy.

The late Clarence Denton, Medical Director of Ives Laboratories, who had worked closely with us on the study, suggested that Ives would seek labeling for use of "Isordil when combined with hydralazine" to reduce mortality in heart failure. It seemed a reasonable thing to do. It would allow Ives to advertise its use, and it would educate physicians on how to use the drugs. He and his staff prepared what was called a "Paper New Drug Application (NDA)". Such an application was different from the usual NDA, which is customarily based on a study previously submitted to the FDA and then approved as a prelude to submission for final approval. V-HeFT had not been a company-sponsored study. The FDA had not been consulted. The company was submitting a document based on the literature—in this case, primarily the *New England Journal of Medicine* paper, supplemented with all our prior published data. Based on these data, the company would ask to have the approved labeling of their drug altered to reflect the new indication.

We approach the FDA

The FDA was more difficult than I expected. Its biostatisticians re-an-
alyzed our data and concluded that the P value was 0.093 rather than 0.046
because we had chosen to adjust our findings for baseline inequalities in
the groups, a practice that has now become standard. The adjustment was
not, however, identified in our analysis plan. Furthermore, we had elected
not to combine the two treatment arms for analysis because they did not
exhibit similar effects. To the FDA, this also justified a penalty on our
p-value. Their re-analysis led to a doubling of the P value, thus meaning
that chance alone could have caused the difference in mortality nearly 1
in 10 times. The benefit of the treatment was no less (a 28% overall reduction in mortality), but now the confidence in that effect was modestly
reduced. Was it enough to invalidate the results? Certainly not.

As described below, the patent office subsequently approved our
patent application for the drug combination as a method for reducing
mortality in heart failure. They were convinced of the significance of
our data. But it was not enough for the FDA, who denied Ives Laboratories' request to re-label the drug, stating that they did not choose to relax
their usual statistical requirements. The FDA stated that since the drugs
are available for any physician who wants to prescribe them, relabeling
was not essential.

The problem, of course, was that only the well-informed physicians—notably those that participated in V-HeFT—became common
prescribers.

A patent application

Another opportunity arose quite unexpectedly. Shortly after completion of V-HeFT, I was called by a lawyer from the CIBA Corporation
which had provided the hydralazine that we used in V-HeFT. Lawyers,
of course, are always aware of intellectual property issues and he was
no exception. He reported to me that he had in fact developed a patent application in which I was the patent holder based upon the results

of V-HeFT, and identifying the combination of isosorbide dinitrate and hydralazine as an effective treatment to reduce mortality from heart failure. He had taken this patent application to upper management at CIBA to encourage their sponsorship of the patent application. They determined, for reasons I will never understand, that this was not an appropriate thing for CIBA to do and therefore rejected the attempt to patent the drug combination. The attorney called to advise me that the application was completed, and he encouraged me to submit it myself.

I recognized that I was an employee of both the University of Minnesota and the Veterans Administration, with which I had a part-time appointment. Any personal patent application would need to be cleared by these employers. I therefore approached the V.A. and was informed that since they had no means of commercializing products, they would waive their potential ownership and involvement in the patent application, even though the work had been done under a V.A. grant. I approached the University of Minnesota and pointed out that all the work in V-HeFT had been performed in V.A. hospitals and not at the University. They agreed that the University had no claim on the patent.

There was precedence to this patent idea. Shortly after arriving at the University of Minnesota in 1974, a new colleague, Marvin ("Bucky") Bacaner, learned that sodium nitroprusside was being marketed as Nipride based upon my early observations of its efficacy. He pointed out to me that I could have gotten a "use" patent—that is, a patent on the *application* of the drug, even though the drug was old and not patentable. If I had patented this observation, he pointed out, I would now be receiving royalties for the sale of this drug.

"It was too late," I said, since the drug company's perusal of my records at the V.A. Hospital in Washington, D.C. that led to its submission and approval by the Food and Drug Administration had occurred years before. I decided I should go forward with the isosorbide dinitrate-hydralazine patent to protect our discovery. I sought out a patent lawyer in Minneapolis who took the application and submitted it on my behalf. It was ultimately published and allowed: U.S. Patent No. 4,868,179,

Method of Reducing Mortality Associated with Congestive Heart Fail-
ure using Hydralazine and Isosrbide Dinitrate.

Perhaps I should have aggressively pursued a sponsor for this drug combination, but we were deeply involved with further analysis of V-HeFT data and with planning a follow-up trial, V-HeFT II, which was designed to build on what we had learned in V-HeFT. Commercialization would have to wait.

Is everyone the same?

One of the often underappreciated truths of clinical trials is that a statistically significant favorable effect does not mean that everyone in the trial benefits comparably. After all, the result in a large trial represents the *average* response in what is often a heterogeneous population. Is it possible to examine the data to determine if the benefit of a drug differs among subpopulations in the study?

After the overall results have been reported, it has become standard practice in trials to explore subsets of the study population to examine the magnitude of benefit of the intervention. Such an exercise is often referred to as "post hoc" since it is an analysis carried out after the data have been collected and analyzed. Because the various subgroups analyzed have not been individually randomly assigned to receive the treatments being compared in a study, the results of such a post-hoc analysis can be used only to generate a hypothesis about a responsive or non-responsive subgroup. Is there a gender difference, or an age difference, or a difference based on some measure of the severity of the disease being treated?

After publishing the overall findings in V-HeFT, we dutifully explored subgroups of our study population. Gender is usually a prominent subgroup for analysis, but all our patients were men. We looked at age groups, different weights, varying severity of disease, different blood pressures, different underlying cardiac diseases causing heart failure, different kidney function. All the subgroups appeared to respond similarly. That is the usual goal of such an analysis—to demonstrate that the treatment works equally well in everyone. We published this conclusion in *Circulation*.

Would Sam Farber have benefitted from this therapy? Had he been examined in the interval between leaving the hospital after recovery from his MI and his readmission with terminal heart failure six months later, a diagnosis of heart failure probably could have been made. Based on our analysis of V-HeFT, his subsequent deterioration could have been prevented.

We did not examine racial background in our analysis of V-HeFT. It was not really an acceptable thing to do in the 1980s. Racial distinction was a sensitive issue. It was also fraught with the difficulty of defining race in a mixed-race population. We didn't really suspect (although in retrospect we should have) that racial background could be a factor in the response to drug therapy. Most clinical trials had been carried out in predominantly white populations, because those were the patients who usually volunteered. So in previous trials not enough black patients, however they might be identified, were studied to form a useful subgroup. It is true that our V.A. population included a substantial number of black men, but we disregarded that distinction in our subgroup analysis.

Years later we would come to appreciate the error of that omission.

CHAPTER IX
Structure Vs. Function

Left ventricular stroke volume, cardiac output, filling pressure, ejection fraction, blood pressure and vascular resistance are all measures of the function of the left ventricle and the arteries. They tell us something about the effectiveness of the heart's contraction and the tone of the walls of the arteries. A powerful heart contraction increases cardiac output. So does an increase in filling pressure. Heightened vascular tone results in an elevated blood pressure. If function of the heart was key to heart failure, as suggested by our Frank-Starling curves, then correcting the functional abnormality with vasodilator drugs should reverse the disease.

But that did not seem to be the case. With infusion of nitroprusside or oral administration of isosorbide dinitrate and hydralazine, we could restore the Frank-Starling curve to normal; that is, we could normalize the filling pressure and normalize the cardiac output. That made patients feel better, but they were still sick. They were still tired, couldn't exert themselves normally, were limited in their activity, and died prematurely. Correcting the functional abnormality clearly was not an adequate way to restore the patient to good health.

Addressing the problem would require imaging of the heart chambers and walls to evaluate its structure. X-ray was of little value because all it could show was a shadow where the heart resided. This shadow provided no insight as to the size of the various heart chambers or the thickness of the walls of the ventricles, the pumping chambers of the heart.

Ultrasound machines, which generate high frequency sound waves that reflect back to the instrument, are capable of defining the precise dimensions of different tissues and fluids at which the instrument is aimed. Ultrasound machines were beginning to be used for medical diagnosis, and the new field of echocardiography was employing ultrasound to examine the heart. We had acquired in Washington a rather cumbersome early machine and utilized it to examine some of our patients. Their left ventricular chambers were strikingly enlarged.

The traditional view was that enlargement of the left ventricle in heart failure resulted from more blood left in the ventricle after its contraction. Since the heart did not empty very well because of its impaired function, the volume left in the chamber was increased, and the pressure in the chamber before the next beat (the filling pressure) was elevated. Pressure and volume would, of course, be increased in parallel, it was thought. The enlarged chamber, therefore, was viewed as evidence that the heart was utilizing its Frank-Starling mechanism to enhance contractile force as a consequence of increased filling. If that were the case the left ventricle would get smaller when the filling pressure fell in response to our vasodilator treatment.

Using ultrasound, we tried to track the chamber dimension as heart function improved during infusion of nitroprusside in a group of patients. To our surprise, as the filling pressure fell, the left ventricle got bigger, not smaller in some patients. What a paradox! A lower filling pressure in diastole should be associated with a smaller chamber. When you let air out of a balloon, the pressure in the balloon falls and the balloon gets smaller. It's simple physics.

Why would the chamber enlarge? It could only be because we had changed the compliance of the ventricle—the relationship between its pressure and volume. Perhaps the ventricle had been stiff, on a steep pressure:volume relationship (Figure VII-5). If nitroprusside relaxes the heart muscle as well as the smooth muscle in the arteries, then a fall in filling pressure could reflect, at least in part, an improvement in compliance or a reduction in left ventricular stiffness.

Why was the ventricle stiff? Certainly structural changes in the wall of the left ventricle (scar tissue or fibrosis or collagen) could make the heart stiff. But clearly some of the stiffness was functional since it could be acutely reversed with nitroprusside. Study of the factors that control stiffness or compliance of the left ventricle is a focus of current interest in some laboratories.

Our studies showed that function of the heart could be independent from structure. The enlarged left ventricular chamber in heart failure was not necessarily a result of a higher filling pressure, or a functional disorder. It had to be structural, because when we improved function and lowered filling pressure the heart could get bigger, not smaller. And its chamber never returned to a normal size, even if the filling pressure was reduced to normal. Yes, improving function might make patients feel better, but perhaps their long-term outcomes were dependent on structure.

This message was subsequently brought home to me by the results of V-HeFT. We had studied two separate vasodilator drug regimens. Both had been chosen based on their ability to improve the function of the heart by reducing impedance and enhancing left ventricular emptying. In short term studies these drugs normalized the Frank-Starling curve. But long-term, one drug improved outcome and the other did not. Functional improvement was obviously not an adequate explanation for the improved survival in the patients treated with isosorbide dinitrate and hydralazine. So what was it?

We had been disregarding structure. Cardiac output and filling pressure tell us nothing about the underlying structure. When dealing with acutely ill patients, it was function that counted. If the cardiac output was too low, the patient may be in shock. If the resistance to flow was too high, the patient might have hypertension. If the filling pressure was too high, he or she might have heart failure. These were functional abnormalities. Structure of the heart and arteries was harder to measure and had largely been disregarded. Indeed, ejection fraction had been viewed as a measure of function. It was assumed to be dependent on the force or power of the contraction.

Our V-HeFT data showed that the drugs that improved outcome—isosorbide dinitrate and hydralazine—produced long-term improvement in ejection fraction, whereas prazosin did not. This was a mystery since both regimens were vasodilators that improved function. If function was improved, why did one regimen increase ejection fraction but not the other?

Like all solutions to knotty problems, once the answer became apparent we wondered why it hadn't previously been recognized. Ejection fraction is more than function. It is critically dependent on volume in the heart, which was determined by structure. If the left ventricular chamber enlarges so that its volume is increased while the stroke volume is constant, then the ejection fraction will fall (Figure IX-1).

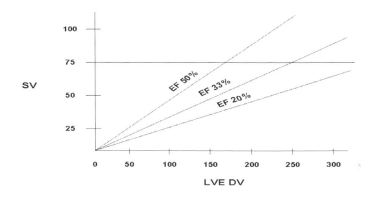

Figure IX – 1

Graph depicting the relationship between stroke volume (SV)—the blood pumped by the left ventricle in each beat—and the ejection fraction (EF)—the fraction of blood in the left ventricle (LV) ejected with each beat. The EF is reduced primarily because of a rise in the end diastolic volume in the LV, not necessarily because of a decline in SV.

It wasn't really that the function of the heart was worse—since the stroke volume and cardiac output might be the same—but that the structure had changed. The chamber had enlarged. The body did not require more cardiac output or blood flow, which would have resulted if the ejection fraction had remained normal. Ejection fraction was in fact a guide to structure of the heart. So perhaps the benefit of isosorbide dinitrate and hydralazine on ejection fraction was not primarily because it improved function, but rather because it improved structure by inhibiting or reversing the enlargement of the chamber.

The myocyte

The major structural element of the heart is the myocyte, or muscle cell, which does the work of contracting. Enlargement of the heart muscle does not result from increasing the number of muscle cells, but from enlargement of the ones we have. In fact, we probably have nearly as many myocytes when we are born as we will ever have. Myocytes disappear during life, but not many new ones are formed.

As shown in Figure III-2, the myocyte is composed of contracting elements called sarcomeres. The vertical lines in this electron microscopic picture of a dog myocyte represent individual sarcomeres that make up the contracting element of the myocyte. When the myocyte enlarges (hypertrophies), as it does with exercise training or with hypertension in response to an increased workload, the myocyte grows new sarcomeres. That growth process involves genes and signaling processes that are now the focus of research efforts in many basic laboratories around the world. Where these new sarcomeres are laid down in the myocyte determines whether the heart muscle thickens or lengthens, and that is an important determinant of how the structure of the heart muscle changes in response to a work load such as high blood pressure, or an injury like myocardial infarction.

What we had not appreciated in the late 1970s, when we were preparing to initiate V-HeFT, was that the structure of the heart could be altered in the absence of stresses that we knew about. Of course, high blood pressure puts a burden on the heart, which responds by thickening the myocytes. Leaky or obstructing valves in the heart can burden the heart and cause muscle cells to grow. Even long-distance runners enlarge their hearts because of the burden of prolonged exercise, but these changes reverse when the repetitive exercise is discontinued.

When observations were made after AMI, however, it became apparent that in some individuals the heart begins to enlarge over time for no known reason. Working in Boston, Marc and Janice Pfeffer created myocardial infarctions in rats by tying off a coronary artery. In surviving animals with large areas of muscle damage, the heart progressively enlarged over time and the animals died prematurely.

The dog laboratory

Was this progressive structural remodeling an explanation for Sam Farber's slowly progressive deterioration in 1956?

I decided to move to the animal laboratory where I could monitor experimental subjects more carefully than in the clinical environment. The laboratory dog, purchased from suppliers that collected them from pounds before they were euthanized, was an ideal experimental subject because they were large enough to allow careful study of heart function and structure. Animal rights groups hadn't yet mobilized to block animal research conducted to better understand human disease. The dogs became involuntary participants in our research and in return were saved from the executioner and gained the friendship and attention of our canine-loving laboratory personnel. We haven't yet as a society come to grips with if or how animals are to be bred or used for medical research, but in the early 1970s, unclaimed and unwanted pound dogs were routinely available for our studies.

I needed a way to produce localized myocardial damage. But I didn't want to tie off a coronary artery and produce an infarct similar to that in man. That would require opening the dog's chest and introducing a whole new set of surgical complications. Furthermore, the dog's coronary circulation is very different from that in humans. Occlusion of a coronary artery in the dog often does not produce an infarct, and certainly not one of predictable size.

I turned instead to a method based on previous observations that patients subjected to electrical defibrillation for cardiac arrest often exhibit localized necrosis or scar formation in the heart. These scars represent electrical burns from the current passed through the paddles on the chest wall. We reasoned that we could produce more localized injury with less electrical current if we passed the electrical activity directly inside the heart.

With painstaking trial-and-error over a period of months, Peter Carlyle (my animal laboratory coordinator) and I developed a protocol using a wire passed into the heart through a catheter advanced into the left ventricle, much like I had used in the patients. We then delivered repetitive electrical shocks across the heart muscle between the wire and a paddle on the chest wall of the anesthetized dog. The result was a well-localized scar in the left ventricle that seemed not to bother the dogs after they awoke from the anesthesia. Although the filling pressures increased acutely, just as it did in the first few hours after AMI, the pressures fell within a day. The dogs returned to their usual activity without apparent distress.

When we monitored the animals over the following weeks, however, the ventricle began to enlarge and heart failure appeared after a few months. This occurred without any new initiating event.

We had succeeded in producing an animal model that appeared to replicate the course of Sam Farber's illness after his MI. Enlargement of the heart and worsening heart function months after a heart attack isn't necessarily the result of some further damage to the heart muscle or some mysterious infection, as my mentors at the Beth Israel Hospital had tried to claim in 1956. It may be a progressive process somehow initiated by the original damage. We had once again succeeded in translational research in the opposite direction—taking a clinical observation and translating it to the animal laboratory.

What could be causing this structural change? Growth of myocytes was being studied in several laboratories, often using isolated myocytes grown in cell culture. In the intact heart, myocytes are exposed to stresses such as elevated blood pressure during contraction, which can make them grow. In culture, however, the myocyte is a passive cell doing no work. In these isolated cell studies, when certain hormones, like norepinephrine and angiotensin, were added to the cell culture, the cells grew by forming new sarcomeres. Synthesis of sarcomeres—the building blocks of myocyte enlargement or hypertrophy—was therefore influenced by more than the work load of the heart. They could respond to hormonal stimulation.

The role of hormones

We suspected that heart failure was accompanied by sympathetic nervous system activation, which is mediated by norepinephrine, and kidney activation, which leads to elevated angiotensin levels. Precisely why these hormonal systems are activated was unclear, but the perception was that this was a response to reduced cardiac function. As humans evolved, the biggest threat to survival was trauma. Being gored by a mammoth was a life-threatening experience. Loss of blood volume would lead to a fall in cardiac output and a fall in blood pressure that would impair blood flow to the brain. Brain function was necessary to recognize the importance of finding a cave as shelter from further assaults. Release of norepinephrine and angiotensin from the nerve endings and from the kidney would support the blood pressure and brain blood flow by constricting arteries in the body but not in the brain. If the primitive human recovered by regaining the depleted blood volume over time, the nervous system response would be turned off. It was an acute protective mechanism for short-term support of the circulation.

But if the same system is activated in response to heart damage that also lowers blood pressure, and if the vasoconstriction induced by the nervous system activation further impairs the function of the heart, then a vicious circle of progressive impairment of the circulation may be initiated. Furthermore, if the activation of norepinephrine and angiotensin also induces structural heart changes that have long-term adverse consequences, then we might have a fuller understanding of what happened to Sam Farber (Figure IX-2).

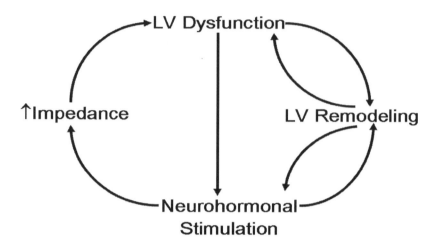

Figure IX-2

Proposed mechanism of worsening heart failure. An initial impairment in heart function (LV Dysfunction) elicits stimulation of the sympathetic nervous system and the renin-angiotensin system (neurohormonal stimulation). This leads to an increase in impedance, which further impairs heart function and also contributes to structural changes (LV remodeling).

But the pattern of response could vary. I learned that from Helen Cleary, a woman who arrived in the coronary care unit of the University of Minnesota Hospital shortly after I assumed my new position as chief in 1974. Helen's arrival was dramatic. She was transferred by ambulance from her community hospital in southern Minnesota, along with her husband Frank, 24 hours after being admitted with what the local doctors called an acute MI. She was on a stretcher sitting bolt upright. Despite an oxygen mask, she was panting for breath and sweating profusely—clearly suffering from acute pulmonary edema. What was particularly striking, besides her life-threatening condition, was her young age. She was 45 years old, even younger than my mother when she had suffered her heart attack. Frank was stunned by the whole episode.

A clinical crisis

I examined Helen as she came through the door of the CCU. She was intensely vasoconstricted and I could feel no pulses in her cold, moist arms or legs. I couldn't measure blood pressure with an arm cuff. But by that time I knew that the blood pressure within her arteries would be considerably higher, especially because she was sitting up and talking to us—evidence that her brain was getting blood flow. The electrocardiogram accompanying her showed a loss of electrical forces across the entire front wall of the heart. She appeared to have an extensive myocardial infarction involving the anterior or front wall of the left ventricle, quite similar to Sam Farber's18 years before.

While the medical residents and staff were administering the usual therapeutic approaches, I pondered my options. In my previous life at the V.A. Hospital in Washington we would have rushed our monitoring equipment to the bedside to document the problem and intervene with appropriate therapy, probably nitroprusside. But no such equipment was yet available at the University Hospital, and nitroprusside had never been used there. I had transferred all my equipment to the V.A. Hospital several miles away. I also had not hired any technical help for clinical studies at the University. Susan Ziesche and Joe Franciosa were at the V.A. How was I to deal with this critically ill young woman with a condition I knew we could help, but without the means?

I would have considered using nitroprusside, but none was available at the University because it had to be prepared from powdered chemical. My new research nurse, Susan Ziesche, had just been trained to prepare it and administer it at the V.A., so I called and asked her to come quickly. When she arrived, Helen's condition had not improved very much. The staff was trying to find a vein for IV access. We had no way to know her blood pressure, and I was hesitant to administer nitroprusside without monitoring it, since the drug can sometimes cause a precipitous fall. I told Susan to administer a dose of isosorbide dinitrate, asking Helen to chew it for quicker action. I hoped that the vasodilator effect of this nitrate, which we had just documented in Washington, would tide Helen over until we could deal with her more effectively.

I ran back to my office to deal with an administrative crisis. Five minutes later Susan appeared in my office.

"I can't give the nitrate," she announced, unfurling the paper insert included with every bottle of medication. "It says the drug should never be given to patients with acute myocardial infarction."

I was annoyed at her failure to follow my orders, but appreciated her independent spirit. We were about to break with tradition. I knew it, but Susan had yet to learn it. Conventional wisdom and recommendations were no longer viable. My new research fellow, Jay Mehta, was quick to grab the isosorbide dinitrate and rush to the bedside to administer it. When I arrived at the bedside 10 minutes later, Helen was breathing comfortably. Her arms and legs had warmed and her sweating had stopped. She managed a weak smile—and so did Frank. Needless to say, we continued intermittent administration of the nitrate and nitroprusside was never needed.

Nothing surprised us about this acute episode. Helen had a large infarct that impaired the pumping ability of her heart. This impairment was aggravated by the intense vasoconstriction that raised her impedance. The ventricle's failure to empty adequately had led to blood backing up in the lungs, resulting in pulmonary edema. The nitrate had pooled blood in the veins to relieve the congestion and had modestly lowered impedance to allow better emptying of the heart. Nitroprusside might have been even more effective, but the nitrate had worked.

I wished I had known that in 1957 when I was treating Sam Farber.

Helen's course after this acute episode, however, was not typical. She never really recovered adequate heart function. We tried her on a number of experimental medications aimed at relaxing the arteries or stimulating the heart, but none significantly improved her poor cardiac function. She would go home for a few weeks but invariably return with worsening heart failure. She was accompanied by Frank the first few times, and Frank was always remarkably considerate.

At one point, however, Frank failed to accompany her. When I asked about him, Helen began sobbing. Frank had left her and moved in with another woman, who happened to be one of Helen's best friends. Illness can have its dire consequences—or perhaps Frank's affair preceded her illness. During Helen's last few months, I felt that I might be the only one who really cared.

Heart structural remodeling

We had begun to recognize that a gradual enlargement of the left ventricle was the usual response in patients who did not quickly recover after an acute MI. We could now document that with echocardiography, the ultrasound technique that allowed visualization of the chambers of the heart. We had produced the same sequence of events in our dog model of myocardial damage. An enlarged, dilated left ventricle was what we would expect to find in a patient that developed persistent heart failure after an MI. That probably accounted for the downhill course of Sam Farber. This was the process that we eventually began calling "re-modeling", and which accounted for the fall in ejection fraction.

But Helen's left ventricle did not enlarge. The filling pressure was high, but the chamber was small. It was stiff. The scar in her left ventricle in the area of the infarction was not accompanied by enlargement of the rest of the left ventricle. She couldn't generate an adequate cardiac output because her end-diastolic volume was low despite the high diastolic pressure, and her contraction was limited by the large scar. It would have been labeled today as HFpEF. The problem was more the heart's filling than it's contraction. The heart was too stiff to allow normal filling with blood before each heart beat.

We didn't know how to treat it in 1975 and we still don't know how to treat it today. Had Helen's illness occurred 10 years later, she would have been placed on a transplant list to receive a donor heart.

Are women different from men?

It was no accident that my first case of post-MI stiff heart occurred in a woman. As we have come to appreciate in recent years, women are for more likely than men to enlarge their heart muscle mass with a small chamber than a large chamber. This difference is likely due to the instruction the myocyte receives to enlarge. If new sarcomeres—the building blocks within each muscle cell—develop lengthwise in the muscle, the cell will lengthen and the chamber will enlarge. If, on the other hand, the sarcomeres develop transversely to thicken the muscle, the chamber wall will thicken but the chamber will not enlarge. Women are more prone to thickening, men to enlarging. The basis for this gender difference is not yet understood.

I was convinced that Sam Farber's heart chamber had enlarged, and that it was a condition that we were beginning to think we could prevent with drug therapy.

Joe Franciosa had been recruited to Philadelphia to become chief of cardiology at the V.A. Hospital. To replace him as chief of research at the Minneapolis V.A., I invited Gary Francis, who had been on the staff of the Hennepin County Medical Center in Minneapolis, to move to the V.A. I recognized that Gary's intellectual curiosity and dedication to improving patient care were similar to my own. In the subsequent years of collaboration, I came to appreciate not only his commitment, but also his scholarship. He read and retained everything of pertinence that was published. He was an effective partner as we challenged traditional thinking.

We decided to study the hormonal responses in our heart failure patients as a clue to whether activation of these systems might be playing a role in progression. There were three vital systems that we thought might be involved: the sympathetic nervous system through the hormone norepinephrine, the renin system through the hormone angiotensin, and the anti-diuretic hormone system through the action of vasopressin. Norepinephrine was released from sympathetic nerve fibers through the body, angiotensin had its origin primarily in the kidney, and vasopressin was secreted from the brain. All these hormones could be measured in blood. The measurements became the responsibility of Ada Simon and her biochemistry laboratory.

The concept was less than perfect. When the sympathetic nervous system is activated by a fall in blood pressure, the nerve endings release norepinephrine, which is the substance that causes blood vessels to constrict and stimulate the myocytes or heart muscle cells to grow. These effects are exerted locally, right at the nerve endings. The norepinephrine that gets into the blood is referred to as "spillover". It may serve as a marker for activation, but the norepinephrine in the blood itself does not actually produce the effect. So it is a pretty indirect measure of nervous system activation.

Angiotensin is another story. The response of the kidney to a reduced blood pressure or blood flow is to secrete renin, which itself does not exert any effect but rather serves to facilitate the formation of angiotensin from a protein produced in the liver. The laboratory test used was a measure of "renin activity". Instead of measuring the level of angiotensin in the blood, it measured the ability of the renin in the blood to generate angiotensin during a period of incubation. So the result was reported as renin activity, the amount of angiotensin generated per hour in the laboratory. Now it is also possible to measure pre-formed angiotensin in blood, but it is a laborious and meticulous procedure that Ada Simon mastered some years later.

Angiotensin is a powerful blood vessel constrictor and also stimulates heart muscle cells to grow. Vasopressin is released from the brain in response to the blood becoming too concentrated—that is, there is not enough water in the blood. The scientific term is osmolality. When osmolality rises, the brain senses it, increasing secretion of anti-diuretic hormone, or vasopressin, which stimulates the kidney to reabsorb or conserve water. Since vasopressin is also a potent blood vessel constrictor, its release can also increase impedance.

Our hypothesis, therefore, was that norepinephrine, angiotensin, vasopressin, or perhaps all three were contributing not only to the blood vessel constriction in heart failure, but also to the structural abnormality of the left ventricle. In addition, I had become interested in a possible protective role of a vasodilator hormone, nitric oxide, normally released from the inner lining of the arteries. Could deficiency of this substance (identified at the time by future Nobel Prize winners) be contributing to vasoconstriction and structural changes?

I had a team working on each hormone system, much like the teams working with me at the Washington V.A. Hospital a decade earlier. But at that earlier time, the teams were working on disparate processes involving the kidney, the liver and the heart. Now we were all working on one disease process, one "silo" of the health care delivery system. An outstanding group of young cardiologists in my program were contributing to the effort. Along with Gary Francis were Ken McDonald from Dublin, Barry Levine from New York, Maria Teresa Olivari from Milan, Steve Goldsmith from Ohio, Spencer Kubo from New York and Gordon Pierpont from Washington. Our group of young investigators, all dedicated to solving the problem of heart failure, established the University of Minnesota as the premier center in the country for the study of this condition.

Despite the obvious deficiencies of these assays, they turned out to be remarkably helpful. When we measured the blood levels of these hormones in our patients with heart failure and compared them with the levels of hormones in their spouses (an effort to find a control group of comparable age and living conditions), the levels were strikingly higher in the patients than in their spouses. Furthermore, and quite dramatically, the higher the levels the sicker were the patients, and the shorter their life expectancy. We published these observations in the *New England Journal of Medicine* in 1984 and it has become one of the most widely cited articles in the field of cardiology.

So our hypothesis was that activation of these hormonal systems plays a critical role in constricting the arteries that increase the impedance load on the damaged heart and reduces its function. But this activation also may be a contributor to the structural changes in the heart that occur over time and may contribute to progression of the disease. This structural progression we now refer to as remodeling and would become a major focus of future research efforts (Figure IX-2). Whether the hormonal activity served merely as a marker for the severity of disease or contributed directly to the remodeling was still to be clarified. It was still uncertain whether the remodeling could be considered a "compensatory" event—one that could help the heart— or a harmful event that hastened its failure. Whether we could intervene to inhibit the process was still unproved. We had many questions to address.

Inhibiting cardiac structural remodeling

Our canine model of electrical shock-induced myocardial injury provided us the opportunity to address some of these questions. If the process could be clarified and its role understood, I reasoned, the rationale for attempting to inhibit it might become apparent. If the structural remodeling protected the function of the heart after damage to the muscle, then it would be inappropriate to try to block the process. If, on the other hand, it was contributing to the downhill spiral that Sam Farber had experienced, perhaps the therapeutic goal would be to block the remodeling.

Of course, we now knew— thanks to our no-name nitroprusside trial and to V-HeFT— that nitroprusside administered acutely, and isosorbide dinitrate and hydralazine administered chronically, could alter the course of the disease. Was the benefit of these drugs related to inhibition of the structural remodeling process? We had to turn to an animal model to clarify it. We designed a series of experiments carried out in our dog model by Ken McDonald.

We needed a way to precisely measure the heart enlargement over time. Fortunately, the University had recruited a bright young magnetic resonance expert, Kamil Ugurbil, who was dedicated to establishing an investigative program in this discipline. MRI is still the gold standard for precise measurement of structure because of its faithful representation of successive slices of three-dimensional organs. After completion of an imaging study of the heart, one can visually stack the individual slices together and accurately calculate the volume of the muscle and the volume of the chamber.

Since MRI machines are very expensive, the initial work was performed after-hours using the clinical machine housed in the Radiology Department. Ken would put the sedated dogs on a stretcher, cover them with a sheet and wheel them into the X-ray unit where patients in the waiting room might not notice that they were long-eared with unusually hairy faces. Their presence in the waiting room rarely caused any visible response.

The studies were very successful. By three months after the electrical injury to the dogs' heart muscle, the overall mass of the heart muscle had increased, thus confirming hypertrophy. At the time the animals were euthanized some months later, Ken isolated the myocytes from these hearts and demonstrated microscopically that the individual heart cells had enlarged, mostly by lengthening. Even more importantly, the chamber of the left ventricle had enlarged (remodeling). When we measured ejection fraction, it had fallen—and it continued to fall progressively until the end of the follow-up period. Clearly, remodeling had been initiated by a single insult months before, but it had become a progressive process leading to declining function, which really reflected structural remodeling.

We now understood better the unfortunate course of Sam Farber. It had required taking the lives of animals, but we rationalized that by knowing we had actually prolonged their lives, which otherwise would have been terminated in the pounds months earlier. These dogs unwittingly made a major contribution to scientific knowledge.

Was the heart muscle remodeling somehow protective? Was it an appropriate response to damage of the heart muscle? Was it a response designed to help the dog cope with stresses after localized damage to the muscle?

If we could produce the scar and block the remodeling, we could test whether the remodeling was helping to support heart function. Based on our clinical experience with isosorbide dinitrate and hydralazine, and subsequently with angiotensin converting enzyme (ACE) inhibitors (see Chapter 10), we decided to intervene with drug treatment in the dogs after electrical damage to the heart muscle. As in our clinical trials, we randomly assigned some dogs to receive a nitrate drug—much like isosorbide dinitrate—or an ACE inhibitor, starting the day after the muscle was damaged. We had the pills administered by an independent animal technician so that Ken would not know which dogs were treated and which were left alone.

After three months, the animals were re-studied in the MRI machine. The pills had significantly inhibited the hypertrophy of the heart muscle and the structural remodeling that enlarged the chamber. The remodeling process could be blocked.

We then undertook exercise testing in these dogs by running them on a treadmill until they fatigued and became short of breath. The animals whose remodeling was blocked by the drugs ran just as long (or longer) than the animals whose hearts had remodeled. There was no evidence that remodeling was protective. It appeared to be an unwanted structural complication after myocardial injury. We now had a rationale for blocking the process, and we had drugs that appeared to be effective.

We even studied an alpha blocker like prazosin, the vasodilator that failed to produce long-term benefit in V-HeFT. As noted briefly in the last chapter, the drug lowered blood pressure but did not block remodeling in the clinical trial. The drug also did not block remodeling in the dog. Translation worked in reverse. A clinical observation had been confirmed in the animal laboratory.

The purpose of animal research, from the standpoint of a clinical investigator, is to demonstrate scientific principles and possibilities. It can never replace studies in patients, because disease processes and responses to interventions may be entirely different in humans. Our animal studies, however, informed us about the mechanisms of our observations and confirmed that we were onto something important.

But the real work lay ahead—to further document that an intervention to inhibit remodeling improved outcome in patients with heart failure, and to find an optimal drug regimen to accomplish this. We now understood why Sam Farber had been readmitted with severe heart failure months after his MI. We now had some insight as to how he could have been treated to prevent his deterioration. But our data were inadequate to change the way patients were being treated. The FDA had not accepted the isosorbide dinitrate-hydralazine data and nobody was manufacturing or marketing the drug combination. We had work to do to confirm these observations and to bring them into clinical practice.

CHAPTER X
V-HeFT II and the ACE Inhibitor Era

By the time V-HeFT was completed in 1985 and we had reported the favorable effect of the isosorbide dinitrate (ISDN)-hydralazine combination on survival of patients with heart failure, there was growing enthusiasm about the clinical use of inhibitors of angiotensin, the angiotensin converting enzyme inhibitors. Enthusiasm was stimulated both by the concept—a drug that blocks the production of an important natural contributor to blood vessel constriction—and by the fact that these drugs were patented and had potential for robust commercial success. Drug companies were rushing to develop their own effective molecules. The original goal was to develop these drugs for the management of hypertension, which is a condition in which blood vessels are abnormally constricted. The therapy was rational, particularly because some experts thought that hypertension was a condition caused by too much angiotensin coming from the kidney.

Blocking angiotensin

The history of ACE inhibitors is a fascinating story of drug development, which led to a Lasker Award in 1999 for David Cushman and Miguel Ondetti, two chemists who worked for the Squibb Corporation. It started with the demonstration that certain snake venoms exert their toxic effect by raising tissue levels of bradykinin, a potent relaxer of blood vessels that in high levels causes a potentially fatal drop in blood pressure. Bradykinin is a constituent of the blood vessel wall and is normally released in low quantities. Bradykinin levels rise in response to poisonous snake bites because the enzyme that normally rapidly inactivates bradykinin is blocked by the snake venom. The enzyme causing inactivation of normally released bradykinin in the body turned out to be the same enzyme that causes production of angiotensin II. That is, a kininase—which inactivates bradykinin—is the same enzyme as angiotensin-converting enzyme (or ACE), which allows production of angiotensin II (Figure X-1). Thus, snake venom not only prolongs the action of bradykinin, the potent vasodilator, but inhibits the production of angiotensin, which could otherwise counteract the vasodilation.

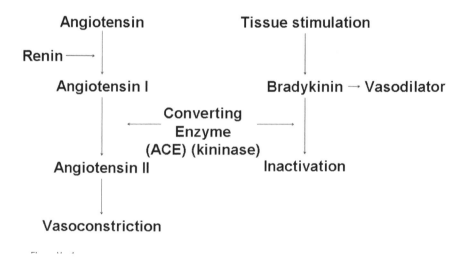

Figure X – 1

The cascade of the renin-angiotensin system and the site of action of angiotensin converting enzyme (ACE) inhibitors. Renin acting on angiotensinogen produces angiotensin I, which is inactive. A converting enzyme (CE), present in tissues, breaks off two amino acids from angiotensin I to form angiotensin II, the active hormone that constricts blood vessels. This CE is the same substance that inactivates bradykinin, a tissue hormone that relaxes blood tissues. ACE inhibitors inhibit the formation of angiotensin II and enhance the activity of bradykinin.

The Squibb Corporation developed a chemical analog of the snake venom that could be given intravenously in doses adequate to block the production of angiotensin II without producing the lethal blood pressure falls of large doses of snake venom. Its goal was to find a new and better treatment for hypertension.

I went to Squibb and presented my evidence that vasodilator drugs improve the function of the failing heart. I proposed that we study this drug in heart failure. They were alarmed at the suggestion, as were a panel of hypertension experts who gathered at Squibb for a consultants' meeting in 1977. To them, heart failure was a disease of the heart. It needed to be treated by making the heart beat more forcefully. There was no rationale, they thought, for treating the blood vessels. The company dismissed my idea and pointed out that lowering the blood pressure was potentially dangerous in patients with heart failure.

Nonetheless, Squibb offered me a small quantity of this precious intravenous medication, and we administered it to a group of patients with heart failure. It was an effective vasodilator and improved heart function, much like nitroprusside and our ISDN/hydralazine combination.

What was strikingly different, however, was that when the drug was infused, the immediate response was dependent on the measured activity of the renin-angiotensin system at the time. Those patients with a big response to the drug had high levels of renin activity, whereas those with little or no response had low levels. In other words, the drug acted through inhibiting the effect of angiotensin rather than directly relaxing the blood vessels, as did ISDN/hydralazine.

We had an attractive concept. The renin system is activated by the poor heart function, angiotensin levels rise to constrict blood vessels, the heart function gets worse, an ACE inhibitor blocks the action of angiotensin, and the patient gets better (Figure X-2).

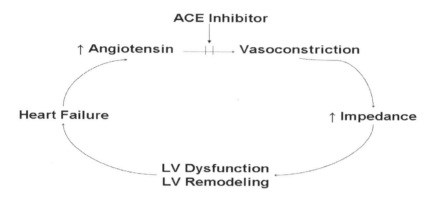

Figure X – 2

By its action to inhibit angiotensin II formation, and perhaps also increase bradykinin, ACE inhibitors reduce impedance and inhibit structural cardiac remodeling, and improve symptoms and survival in heart failure.

What eventually made possible more extensive testing of the hypothesis was that both Squibb and Merck, the two major pharmaceutical companies studying cardiovascular drugs at the time, synthesized compounds that exhibited similar enzyme blocking effects as the snake venom and could be taken orally without destruction in the stomach. These compounds opened the possibility for chronic treatment with a drug that could block the formation of angiotensin II.

The ACE inhibitor era was born.

We and others carried out some preliminary small trials with longer-term administration of an oral ACE inhibitor in patients with heart failure, either captopril from Squibb or enalapril from Merck. The drugs were well-tolerated and they improved heart function. When we finished V-HeFT, the investigators all agreed that our study group should remain intact and take on another project.

This seemed to be the right project. The ISDN and hydralazine combination was effective. Why not compare this drug combination with "the new kid on the block", an ACE inhibitor? I went to Merck, which had developed enalapril—a fairly long acting and effective oral

ACE inhibitor—to suggest that they help support a V.A. Cooperative
Study (V-HeFT II) on the long-term effect of enalapril in patients with
chronic heart failure. By that time the scientific community and the
pharmaceutical industry had concluded that my ideas were not so out-
landish after all.

The V.A. and Merck agreed, the protocol was completed, and the
study was initiated in 1986. We were going to compare the effect on
mortality of our drug combination, ISDN and hydralazine, with the effect of enalapril. No placebo arm was included because the V-HeFT
investigators felt that our first trial had satisfactorily demonstrated that
ISDN/hydralazine was better than placebo, and therefore nobody should
be assigned to take placebo. The investigators no longer had equipoise,
that state in which uncertainty allows you to assign patients to either of
two treatments because you are not certain which is better. Our uncertainty was between ISDN/hydralazine and an ACE inhibitor. We wanted
to find out which was better.

A comparative trial

Not everyone shared our view of the demonstrated effectiveness of
ISDN/ hydralazine. Soon after we began planning V-HeFT II, the National Institutes of Health also decided to do a clinical trial in heart
failure. They also were impressed with the preliminary data on enalapril
and designed a trial to test it in a larger study with far more centers than
we could afford to recruit. I was appointed to the Steering Committee of
that trial to assist in its planning.

They decided on a placebo-controlled trial. I pleaded that treatment
with isosorbide dinitrate and hydralazine should be allowed because
of its demonstrated effectiveness, and that it should be strongly recommended as part of background therapy. I was therefore promoting a
study design that would assess the effectiveness of enalapril added to
background ISDN/HYD treatment compared with ISDN/HYD alone.

The other Steering Committee members did not agree on the
recommendation, but they did vote to allow these drugs in both the

placebo and enalapril-treated arms of the study. After the study was completed, we found that nitrate was commonly employed by the physicians, usually in doses far less than we were advocating, but hydralazine was only rarely used, mostly by those who either participated in V-HeFT or were fully aware of the magnitude of the benefit in V-HeFT. This trial, SOLVD (Studies of Left Ventricular Dysfunction) was therefore designed to determine if enalapril compared to placebo would prolong survival in heart failure when added to standard therapy, which now often included nitrate in addition to diuretic and digoxin.

In retrospect, V-HeFT II was a mistake, not because of the drugs we decided to test, but because of the design of the study. At the time it seemed the right thing to do. In fact, even the current funding effort by the federal government encourages such research under the title "comparative efficacy". The goal was (and is) to document which of alternate possible therapies produces the better outcome. In order to improve efficiency of care, it is reasoned, we need to study different strategies to pick the best "evidence-based therapy".

So what's the matter with studies of comparative efficacy? If we have two possible drug treatments for heart failure why shouldn't we compare them to identify which is better?

It certainly made sense in 1985. We had demonstrated to our satisfaction that the isosorbide dinitrate (ISDN) and hydralazine combination was an effective treatment for heart failure and could both increase survival and improve the function and probably the structure of the left ventricle. Now we had a new class of drugs to compare to the old.

Then why was V-HeFT II a mistake?

We were assuming a uniform response. If we compare two groups in a long-term trial and find that one treatment (Treatment A) reduces mortality more than the other treatment (Treatment B), the usual interpretation is that Treatment A is better than Treatment B. Therefore, everyone should receive Treatment A. That is the philosophy of the government's advocacy for comparative efficacy studies. If the two treatments produce a similar outcome, it would be assumed that the drugs are equally effective and one could be substituted for the other.

But when two drugs appear to work through a different mechanism of action, one can never assume that different patients are responding similarly to the two drugs. One group of patients might respond better to Drug A, and another group of patients might respond better to Drug B. The difference in outcome in the two treatment arms may be related to the proportion of responders to treatment A or to treatment B in the study population.

How might you identify the responder population?

One way is to search the data for possible patient descriptors associated with a good response. But you can only explore the descriptor data collected. If, for example, blue eyes or dark hair are critical genetic traits identifying responders, we couldn't detect them because these traits are not recorded. Self-identified race is recorded, and it may be associated with certain genomic differences that have served as identifiers of geographic family origin, but such genomic identifiers are complicated and not routinely analyzed.

Should we casually assume that an effective treatment in a clinical trial applies to all populations, or are differences in response so prominent that we should confine our assumptions to the population studied? Carried to an extreme such uncertainly can threaten our comfort with so-called "evidence-based medicine".

Could phenotype (description of the disease) rather than genotype (description of the patient's genomic profile) help?

If plasma renin activity predicts the response to an ACE inhibitor, maybe this or other measures of disease mechanism might help to distinguish responders from non-responders. With antibiotics, such a distinction is well understood. One drug might attack gram-positive bacteria and another gram-negative bacteria. Even if the number of patients benefiting in a trial were similar, one would never conclude that the drugs are equal. We do cultures to identify the offending bacteria, and treat with a drug known to attack that bacterium.

With a disease like heart failure, where the mechanism is less clear, a similar benefit from Drug A and Drug B might mistakenly lead to the assumption that the drugs are equal in their effect. But they may not be equal. Some patients may be better on one drug and some on the other. Thus, I have now reached the conclusion that one should never do a comparative trial of one treatment versus another *different* form of treatment in a disease unless one includes a treatment arm in which the two therapies are given together. Two drugs which have an equal effect when given alone might have an *additive* benefit when given together because they are working on two different populations of patients.

Many clinical trialists still fail to recognize this important principle. Our goal in developing therapies for chronic diseases is not to compare one drug to another, but to identify optimal therapy. It is generally pharmaceutical companies who perform comparative trials in order to gain a marketing advantage over their competitors. Such studies do not necessarily serve the scientific community.

A marketing advantage

There was another more subtle problem with V-HeFT II. The playing field for the two drug regimens was not level. Enalapril was supported and marketed by a powerful pharmaceutical company with massive resources. ISDN and hydralazine, on the other hand, were generic drugs with no sponsor and no marketing. Merck was involved in supporting extensive pre-clinical and clinical research with enalapril that attracted widespread attention. Nobody was studying ISDN and hydralazine.

We did not include a placebo arm in V-HeFT II because we felt a moral obligation to provide patients either with the therapy we felt had been previously shown to be effective, or another therapy that might be as effective or even more effective. We did not appreciate how much skepticism would grow over subsequent years with our V-HeFT interpretation. If we had been right in V-HeFT, then everyone should be taking ISDN and hydralazine as therapy for their heart failure. They were not, however, in part because no one was marketing the drug combination, and so physicians were not reminded about it.

Furthermore, the commercially available preparations of hydralazine made it very difficult and cumbersome to administer in the doses we had used in V-HeFT. No one was interested in selling the concept because the two medications were generic and could be bought by prescription for pennies a day. So in retrospect, perhaps we could have justified including a placebo arm in V-HeFT II. And, of course, we should also have included an arm in which enalapril and the ISDN-hydralazine combination were given together. But given the modest sample size that we felt we could recruit in our thirteen V.A. centers, such an expansive protocol was beyond our means.

V-HeFT II was completed in 1990. To this day the results have been difficult to interpret. Were the two treatments equal or were they different? After two years of follow-up, there was a slight difference in survival favoring the group taking enalapril, the ACE inhibitor. At the end of trial, which was the primary end-point for the study, the two treatments were not different from each other, although there was a slight but insignificantly preferential benefit of enalapril.

The mortality curves are displayed in Figure X-3. The p-value for the difference was 0.083, not low enough by traditional criteria to exclude a play of chance, but low enough to suspect that the ACE inhibitor might be more effective than the ISDN/hydralazine. Keep in mind that the study was not adequately powered to demonstrate equivalency of the two treatment arms. All one can do is search for evidence that the two treatment arms are different. Not being different does not necessarily mean equivalence. That is an arcane but vital biostatistical fact. Equivalency is very difficult to prove because you must exclude a difference. A difference is easier to demonstrate because all that is required is to reject the null hypothesis of no difference.

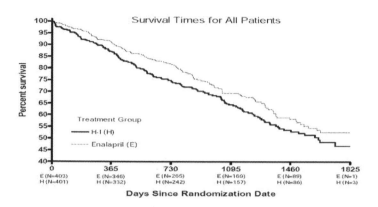

Figure X-3

Survival curves in V-HeFT II. There was a trend for better survival in the patients receiving enalapril than those receiving ISDN/hydralazine. But the overall difference
was not statistically significant.

The results of V-HeFT II were published in the same 1991 issue
of the *New England Journal of Medicine* as the NIH-sponsored SOL-
VD Trial. Both studies were completed about the same time and the
two manuscripts written simultaneously. I was intimately involved in
preparing both papers. I was the senior author of V-HeFT II and wrote
the final manuscript with the consent of our Steering Committee. I was
a member of the SOLVD Steering Committee that contributed to that
publication as well.

The message conveyed by these two companion papers was that
enalapril, the ACE inhibitor, was a valuable life-saving treatment for
heart failure. SOLVD had randomized over 3000 patients equally divid-
ed between placebo and enalapril treatment. The enalapril-treated patients had a 15% lower mortality rate than the placebo-treated patients.
The difference was modest but highly statistically significant because of
the large sample size.

The interpretation of the much smaller V-HeFT II was that it confirmed SOLVD. In V-HeFT II, there were slightly fewer deaths in the
enalapril group than the ISDN/hydralazine group, although the differ-

ence was hardly significant, with only 400 patients in each group. In some reports of the study the fact was disregarded that the control group did not receive placebo but rather ISDN and hydralazine, the effective treatment in V-HeFT I. It was sufficient for the medical profession to conclude that ACE inhibitors were good treatment. ISDN/hydralazine was disregarded, even assumed to be no better than a placebo. Had we included a placebo arm, I am confident the effectiveness of ISDN/hydralazine would have been confirmed.

Differential cardiac remodeling

The ejection fraction data in V-HeFT II were critically important, but often disregarded in the medical community's fascination with survival curves. Both treatments resulted in a sustained increase in ejection fraction, implying that left ventricular structural remodeling had been improved. In fact, during the first year after randomization, the ejection fraction rose more in the ISDN/hydralazine group than in the enalapril group.

To us, the main finding was that both interventions produced a sustained improvement in left ventricular structure, which in V-HeFT was associated with a benefit on survival. Our conclusion was that both therapies apparently worked by inhibiting structural remodeling, and both therapies prolonged survival.

We went so far as to superimpose the survival curves in V-HeFT II onto the survival curves in V-HeFT. We proposed that the superimposition was appropriate because both studies were carried out in the same V.A. medical centers in patients with similar entrance criteria. Therefore their outcome should have been similar. The hypothesis was that the placebo arm in V-HeFT could therefore be used as a hypothetical placebo arm for V-HeFT II. In the superimposed data it was clear that ISDN/hydralazine as well as enalapril produced a striking improvement in survival. ISDN/hydralazine increased survival by an average of 10 months, and enalapril increased it by an average of 16 months.

I had introduced a measurement in V-HeFT II that was not included in V-HeFT. Because of our fascination with the role of hormonal stimulation on the course of heart failure, we collected blood samples in all patients for the measurement of norepinephrine and renin activity at baseline, and we monitored norepinephrine sequentially during follow-up. All the V-HeFT II samples were shipped frozen to Minneapolis where Ada Simon performed the assay.

As we had previously shown in our own small population at the University of Minnesota, elevated levels of these hormones at baseline were powerful predictors of mortality. Enalapril therapy, which inhibits the renin system, also reduced norepinephrine, suggesting that the renin-angiotensin system and the sympathetic nervous system—two of the hormone systems activated in heart failure—are interactive. The benefit of enalapril on remodeling of the left ventricle and on survival could therefore be attributed to its hormonal inhibiting effect.

But what about ISDN/HYD?

It also inhibited remodeling and improved survival, but plasma norepinephrine levels rose, not fell, in the group treated with those drugs. We thought that ISDN/HYD must be operating through a different mechanism not involving the sympathetic nervous system or renin-angiotensin system. But we had no idea what that mechanism was. It was years later that nitric oxide, the end product of ISDN/hydralazine metabolism, would be discovered as a critical factor in vascular and cardiac health. It was clear then, and certainly now, that these drugs were acting though entirely different mechanisms and that comparing efficacy was a flawed strategy.

It's an ACE world

Another trial with enalapril had also been supported by Merck—the Cooperative North Scandinavian Enalapril Survival Study (CONSENSUS). This study was confined to a remarkably sick population of Scandinavians with what is called Class IV heart failure. Class IV heart failure is diagnosed in patients who are so limited by fatigue and shortness of breath that they are unable to carry out any normal life activities. The patients are essentially bed-ridden or chair-ridden, and their life expectancy is very short. Since therapy at that time was limited to digoxin and diuretic, there was little to offer these patients. The Scandinavian investigators suggested to Merck that they would randomize such patients to receive either placebo or enalapril, the ACE inhibitor.

The outcome of this trial surprised even the investigators. Within one year of beginning therapy the mortality rate in the enalapril arm was so reduced compared to the placebo arm that the trial was terminated prematurely by the Data Safety and Monitoring Board, which felt all patients should be offered the superior efficacy of enalapril.

CONSENSUS consisted of an unusual patient population. These patients were quite elderly and their blood pressures were not very well controlled when they entered the trial. Enalapril, which had already been approved as an effective anti-hypertensive agent, lowered the blood pressure as well as strikingly reduced the mortality. This population was not typical of those observed in the U.S. and is now very atypical for a patient population with severe heart failure. Nonetheless, the results of CONSENSUS proved to all skeptics that therapy with an ACE inhibitor could improve outcome in patients with heart failure.

The FDA reviewed the outcome benefit in CONSENSUS and SOL-VD and reached the conclusion that this therapy should be approved for the management of heart failure. Thanks to the marketing efforts of Merck and, subsequently, other pharmaceutical companies that introduced their own ACE inhibitors, these drugs gained widespread use in the management of heart failure. Indeed, guidelines prepared by various organizations advising proper management of heart failure mandated administration of ACE inhibitors. The era of ACE inhibitors was thus in full swing. It was no longer ethical to perform a trial in heart failure without encouraging all patients to take an ACE inhibitor.

The data collected in these two V-HeFT trials taught us so much that was new about this complicated disease that I published a compendium of our findings. I was still sensitized to our failure to pursue the ancillary data in our previous nitroprusside. I was able to generate a modest grant from Merck to organize a retreat where all the investigators would gather to write papers. I hired a couple of talented medical writers to work with us in organizing the manuscripts. We spent a long working weekend on Martha's Vineyard and churned out the rough drafts of a dozen papers that eventually were published as a self-contained supplement to *Circulation*, the official journal of the American Heart Association. Over the years many of my colleagues have referred to this publication as the "Bible of Heart Failure". I had also often been accused by my colleagues of sermonizing on the topics of the mechanisms of heart failure and its treatment. But these were not stories nor beliefs.. This was science, not religion. There was no need to suspend scientific discipline. The data were clear for all to see.

Yet the place of ISDN/hydralazine, the drug combination that started the whole search for new drugs for chronic heart failure, remained controversial and was largely disregarded in the practice of medicine.

CHAPTER XI
Intellectual Property and BiDil

I owned the patent for combined use of ISDN and hydralazine to reduce mortality in heart failure, thanks to the patent office agreeing that we had shown a reduction in mortality, even if the FDA did not. I informally queried a number of large pharmaceutical companies regarding their possible interest in developing and marketing this drug combination, but there were too many downsides. The drugs were generic and could be obtained quite inexpensively. Our protocol in V-HeFT was to administer the drugs four times a day, which was viewed as a serious impediment to patient compliance and marketing. Most companies also perceived that the potential market would be small because of the widespread and growing use of ACE inhibitors to treat heart failure. No one expressed interest until I met Manfred Mosk.

Manfred was a Romanian phenomenon. He had a Ph.D. from a school that I had never heard of. He appeared to know everyone who was politically well-connected, and he confided in me once that his secret ambition was to become American ambassador to Romania. Manfred had founded a small pharmaceutical company that was dedicated to licensing products, primarily those developed at universities, and bringing them to market through the FDA approval process. He expressed great interest in ISDN/hydralazine.

Over a number of months, we met at various meeting sites around the world discussing the prospects. He was gregarious, demonstrative and ebullient. At most of our meetings he reveled in hugging and kiss-

ing me, perhaps a European style that didn't afflict most of my European friends. His company appeared to consist of less than 10 employees,
but he had licensed a powerful drug, adenosine, from friends and colleagues at the University of Virginia. I had no other options. We signed
a licensing agreement in which Medco Research acquired rights to my
patent in return for stock options, royalties and a seat on their Board of
Directors.

Medco Research

My Board involvement was a learning experience. Even before my
first Board meeting, Manfred had resigned from the Board "for personal reasons" that were never discussed. The other Board members were
experienced in finance or pharmaceutical company business so I gained
much insight into the workings of the business and the dedication to
the bottom line. It was clear that the company's orientation, especially
that of the president who had a research background, was to adenosine
products.

Adenosine receptors are involved in a number of biologic processes
related to heart rhythm abnormalities, kidney function, coronary artery
blood flow and even heart failure. Thus I was able to make useful contributions to Board and management issues as they explored various
opportunities with adenosine compounds and with various drugs that
could block the effects of adenosine.

Further development of ISDN/Hydralazine was always a lower priority on the agenda, but the company did pursue the opportunity. The
first order of business was to develop a combination product that contained an appropriate dose of both isosorbide dinitrate and hydralazine.
The company hired a manufacturing company to do the formulation
work and undertake the pharmacokinetic (blood level of drugs) studies
required to show that the formulated combination pill, when taken by a
volunteer, provided the same blood levels as taking the two drugs separately. Establishing such bioequivalence is a rigorous requirement of the
FDA for any newly compounded drug.

The next order of business was to name the drug. A contest was announced for all employees and directors to submit proposals. I sorted through a variety of possible names that would reflect the two components. But Isozine, Nitrazine, Hydralazate and Sorbazate did not slip easily off the tongue. One employee who I did not know came up with the winner: BiDil. It was a perfect fit.

As the name implied, it was composed of two vasodilator drugs, and the name was easy to pronounce and remember. Little did we know that subsequent research would show that hydralazine may not be acting primarily as a vasodilator, but rather as an antioxidant, which I will explain later. At the time, BiDil seemed right. It still does.

It soon became clear that Medco Research was not prepared to invest in a new trial with BiDil. V-HeFT was a small trial (only 186 patients taking ISDN/Hyd) that had been performed a number of years earlier. More recent trials seeking FDA approval had been much larger. Ives Laboratories had already sought approval by the FDA of the ISDN component without success. But Medco's plan was to put together a more persuasive presentation along with the data on the combined tablet, BiDil, and go back to the FDA for approval.

I helped prepare a comprehensive document that reviewed all of our data and laid out a compelling argument for approval of BiDil for heart failure. Our proposal stressed three themes: one, the drugs are known to be safe because of many years of experience using them for other indications; two, the data on effectiveness in heart failure are all consistent with a favorable effect; and three, approval will allow the sponsor to inform doctors about how to use the drug.

The FDA approval process

It is important to explain the FDA approval process for new indications for drugs. Investigational studies of unapproved drugs are conducted through an IND, or Investigational New Drug application. When the sponsor concludes that enough data have been generated they prepare an NDA, or New Drug Application. The FDA is given a limited amount of time to respond to an NDA. It can approve the drug, reject it, or send the application back for more information.

An FDA Advisory Committee of non-FDA experts exists to assist the FDA in decision-making when they feel the issues are not clear. I served as Chairman of the Cardiorenal FDA Advisory Committee from 1979 to 1981 so I was familiar with the process. Although I hoped the FDA would approve our NDA without consulting the Advisory Committee, I realized that the decision was important enough that it would likely require presentation to the Committee, just as it had in 1981 with our first application shortly after I had stepped down as Chairman.

We were notified of the date for the presentation and prepared carefully. Our presentation was scheduled for the afternoon of an all-day meeting in Bethesda, the morning being devoted to a discussion of another heart failure drug, carvedilol (Coreg) sponsored by SmithKline Beecham. My colleagues, including some FDA personnel, were happy to discuss prospects for these two drugs. The general feeling was that SKB's study, which failed to meet its endpoint and had already been disapproved in a previous action, would be unlikely to prevail; whereas Medco Research, with the well-known V-HeFT data base and a sound rationale, would probably succeed.

How wrong we were. Perhaps because of the financial resources of SKB and a polished presentation by their paid consultants, Coreg was recommended for approval by a split vote. I sat through the morning session and concluded that the Advisory Committee had been remarkably tolerant to the company's claims.

The afternoon discussion of BiDil focused not so much on V-HeFT, but on V-HeFT II. Bob Temple, the Director of the Drug Division, was troubled by the benefit of enalapril compared to the drug combination in V-HeFT II (I had previously pointed out that V-HeFT II was ill-advised). Although enalapril did not reduce mortality significantly more than did ISDN/Hyd (that is, the P value was not significant), the magnitude of benefit was 10-15%, similar to the magnitude of benefit of enalapril compared to placebo in SOLVD. Therefore, Temple reasoned, ISDN/Hyd appeared to be no better than a placebo.

Temple was suggesting that V-HeFT had been a fluke, a borderline statistically favorable effect that was a play of chance. He was unmoved by the fact that the magnitude of benefit of ISDN/Hyd in V-HeFT had been closer to 30%, and that the insignificant P value was related primarily to the small sample size that increased the risk of a play of chance.

The supportive data on the ejection fraction, which we thought documented the effectiveness of the drugs, was of no interest to the FDA. They didn't (and couldn't by law) pay attention to end-points that were not measures of benefit to the patient. Ejection fraction or heart remodeling was not, in their view, a measurement that affected patient well-being or survival. Subsequent data have now made it quite clear that it does.

The argument about V-HeFT II mortality findings could not be countered, because we had no additional studies with BiDil. No entity had seen fit to finance another study. It was now no longer possible to do a placebo-controlled trial of BiDil because of the mandate that all patients be treated with an ACE inhibitor. Bob Temple even suggested (outlandishly I thought at the time) that we perform a placebo-controlled trial in Russia where ACE inhibitors were not yet in use. I thought it was ethically indefensible to utilize an underserved population to provide inadequate health care, at least to the group randomized to receive placebo. We were therefore limited to the existing data.

BiDil was turned down by a split vote, with most of the "no's" being registered by biostatisticians and non-physician members of the Committee.

The FDA is not bound by Committee votes but usually follows their recommendations. Nonetheless the FDA agreed to a follow-up meeting with Medco Research and me to discuss ways forward.

After hours of debate in a meeting that extended into the evening, the agency agreed to consider further analysis of V-HeFT to help document the statistical significance of the benefit compared to placebo. But it was clear the agency was going to request another trial, and Medco was not prepared to fund it. At the next Board meeting Medco made the decision to terminate development of BiDil. In July of 1998 I signed a Termination Agreement that returned the intellectual property and the NDA to me.

Shortly afterward, with Medco's future prospects somewhat questionable and a purchase offer on the table, the Board voted to sell the company to King Pharmaceuticals.

NitroMed

Medco was gone and I once again owned the intellectual property. A suitor wasn't long in coming.

This company, NitroMed, was a better fit. It was a research-oriented organization without a marketable product. Its focus was nitric oxide, the substance that we now know is the end product of BiDil treatment. Isosorbide dinitrate is metabolized in the body to a gas, nitric oxide. Nitric oxide is inactivated by oxidative stress, which can be aggravated by continuous isosorbide dinitrate therapy. Hydralazine serves as an antioxidant to protect the nitric oxide from destruction, thus enhancing its effect.

Nitric oxide is a remarkable substance that relaxes the arteries and protects the arteries and heart from the structural changes we had characterized as remodeling. All of this physiology and pharmacology had come from bench research undertaken long after we demonstrated the effectiveness of the components of BiDil.

The importance of nitric oxide (or NO) was emphasized by the Nobel Prize Award Committee, who gave the award in medicine in 1998 to three investigators, Bob Furchgott, Lou Ignarro and Ferid Murad, who identified NO as the vasodilator substance normally released from the inner lining of the arteries,.

NitroMed's interest in nitric oxide placed it firmly into the 21st century. BiDil would give it the potential for a drug that could enhance their financial position and make it a world leader. It was an exciting opportunity. A licensing agreement was signed in January 1999 that transferred the patent rights and NDA to NitroMed in return for stock options, royalties and membership on their Scientific Advisory Board. What I didn't realize at the time was that this agreement would catapult me into racial political issues that I had never faced. As a life-long liberal with what I considered a color-blind approach to social intercourse, I soon found myself facing attack for stances that I thought were rational and balanced.

How much I had to learn.

CHAPTER XII
Black and White

Interest in a possible racial difference in cardiovascular drug therapy response did not start with ISDN and hydralazine, now known as BiDil. It started with ACE inhibitors.

Early studies in patients with hypertension noted that angiotensin converting enzyme (ACE) inhibitors were less effective in lowering blood pressure in hypertensive black patients than in white patients. The reason wasn't fully understood. Some thought that it was because the renin-angiotensin system is less active in black patients compared to white patients, as reflected by a low plasma renin activity. As explained earlier, renin activity is a measure of the ability of the body to synthesize angiotensin, the potent constrictor hormone. ACE inhibitors block its production. The renin system is activated when a person is salt-deprived because one purpose of angiotensin is to conserve salt. Some investigators thought the reduced response to ACE inhibitors was related to greater salt retention in black patients, since salt intake can suppress angiotensin production.

Survival of the fittest

One fascinating hypothesis suggests a Darwinian explanation for the evolution in this country of black people with lower renin activity and salt retention. Since much of the black population in the United States arrived initially on slave ships from Africa, and the conditions on those slave ships were so poor that many died from dehydration, there was a survival advantage to passengers who had a genetic makeup favoring salt retention by the kidney. Thus, the current black population, most of whom were descendants of these slaves, were more likely to have inherited a genomic profile favoring salt retention and low renin activity. An environmental cause related to high salt diet and life style is certainly an alternative or contributing factor.

Regardless of mechanism, the phenomenon of racial differences in response was so well recognized that physicians were advised not to use ACE inhibitors as first-line therapy in black hypertensives. They were advised instead to start with a diuretic, which is particularly effective in black patients, again possibly related to their salt intake or reduced ability of their kidneys to excrete a salt load. Even the labeling of ACE inhibitors by the FDA included a statement that they were less effective in black patients. It was widely accepted, however, that after a diuretic had been administered to relieve the patient of salt retention, the ACE inhibitors were effective in blacks to lower blood pressure, perhaps because the diuretic had stimulated renin production.

ACE inhibitors and race

After completing V-HeFT II, which compared the ACE inhibitor enalapril with our ISDN/Hyd combination, I began wondering about a possible racial difference in response to ACE inhibitors in heart failure. I was surprised that no one had explored this. Perhaps it was because almost all heart failure patients were taking a diuretic for fluid retention, which might have eliminated any racial differences. Perhaps also it was because most of the trials in heart failure had been carried out in a predominantly white population.

In V-HeFT II, which was conducted in VA Hospitals, nearly 30% of our patients identified themselves as black or African-American. Therefore, it seemed to be an ideal opportunity to explore whether race had any apparent impact on the differential response between an ACE inhibitor and ISDN/Hyd.

I discussed the issue with Peter Carson, who had been a fellow at the University of Minnesota and then became principal investigator of our trial center in the V.A. Hospital in Washington, D.C. where I had carried out my early research. We agreed on the approach. We would identify the black and white patients by their self-designated race on our stored data forms and separately analyze the characteristics and outcomes in the two populations.

The weakness in such an approach, of course, is the absence of appropriate randomization. The design of V-HeFT II demanded that treatment with enalapril or ISDN/Hyd be randomly assigned in sequence, regardless of racial designation. When one then evaluates response by race, there is no assurance that randomization led to appropriate assignment to the two therapies. A skewed randomization could certainly have placed sicker patients on one treatment or another by chance. We therefore adjusted all our data for any apparent inequalities in their baseline risk, and we approached the analysis with the idea that we were doing an exploration, not seeking a definitive conclusion. This approach is often called "hypothesis-generating".

Our first look at the data resulted in an "Oh my God!" response from both of us. As shown in Figure XII-1, in the white population enalapril was clearly more effective than ISDN/Hyd, or BiDil. Even in this small population of white patients, the mortality reduction from enalapril compared to ISDN/Hyd was statistically significant. In the even smaller black population there was now no difference in the outcome between enalapril and ISDN/Hyd (Figure XII-1). These data were consistent with our working hypothesis that ACE inhibitors are more effective in white patients than in black patients.

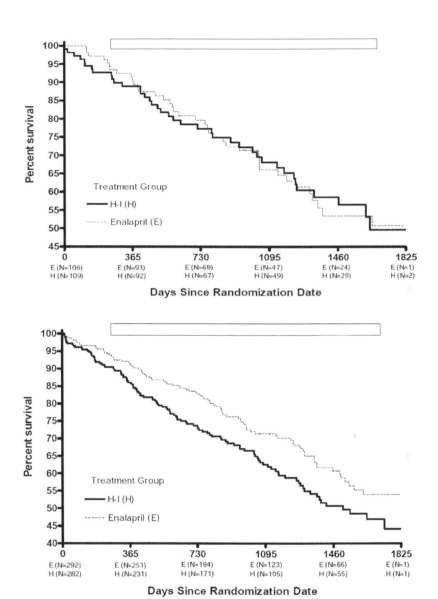

Figure XII-1

Survival curves in V-HeFT II separated into the 215 self-designated black patients (first graph above) and the 574 self-designated white patients (second graph above). Note that the two treatments were equal in the black patients but that enalapril improved survival significantly more than ISDN/hydralazine in the white patients.

BiDil and race

The results of this analysis of V-HeFT II were confounded by the fact that we were comparing enalapril to ISDN/Hyd. If there was a racial difference in response to the BiDil combination it could impact on our perception of a racial difference in ACE inhibitor response. Was there any reason to suspect a racial difference in response to ISDN/Hyd?

This question gets us into what was at the time, and still is, the burgeoning field of nitric oxide (NO) research. We now know, as previously explained, that ISDN exerts its effect by breakdown of isosorbide dinitrate to the gas, NO. This NO is rapidly degraded by oxidative stress. Interestingly—and quite by serendipity when we first put the two drugs together—hydralazine acts as an antioxidant that protects the NO from degradation. Thus, the drug combination can appropriately be referred to as a nitric oxide *donor* or nitric oxide *enhancer*.

Nitric oxide, the discovery of which won the Nobel Prize, is released from the inner lining of the arteries (the endothelium) to relax the artery and protect its structural integrity. In conditions leading to obstruction to arteries, such as heart attacks and strokes, nitric oxide effect is deficient and structural changes occur, such as cholesterol plaque formation and wall thickening. That is a condition we now characterize as "Endothelial Dysfunction".

In the 1990s, laboratories began studying endothelial dysfunction in patients with hypertension and other cardiovascular diseases. Studies were specifically carried out to study endothelial function in different groups, including blacks compared to whites. Those studies consistently showed that black individuals on average exhibited less NO release or activity in response to stimuli that produced a robust effect in whites. If there is less NO available in blacks, then a drug that enhances NO might be particularly effective in blacks. Now there was a basis for the hypothesis that BiDil would be more effective in blacks than in whites. NO has been less well studied in the heart, but it appears that the inner lining of the heart, the endocardium, also is a site of NO release and NO deficiency may contribute to heart structural remodeling.

We had also examined the data from V-HeFT I, in which we compared the outcome in patients with heart failure who received either ISDN/Hyd or placebo. Did the benefit of ISDN/Hyd differ between the white and black patients? It certainly did. The rather small black population exhibited a dramatic 47% lower mortality when taking ISDN/Hyd compared to placebo. The white population showed a small benefit of about 15%, which was not statistically significant.

When Peter Carson and I completed this analysis we were hesitant to publish it. It would be a major and controversial finding based on a retrospective analysis of a prior trial, an exercise that always draws criticism from biostatisticians and clinical trialists who are troubled by data dredged from studies not designed to address the question posed. Furthermore, the overall V-HeFT trials were small, and subdividing the patient population by racial designation made the groups even smaller. Most importantly, it was about race, a sensitive topic in America. Had we found a different response based on gender, body mass index, blood pressure or any other demographic marker, we would have rushed to report it, despite the caveats. But patient selection based on race was widely viewed as discrimination.

There were no other data on ISDN/Hyd to search, but there certainly were data on ACE inhibitors. If we could confirm a differential effect of ACE inhibitors in another heart failure trial, I felt we would have enough confirmation to go forward with publishing our observations.

The CONSENSUS trial comparing placebo to enalapril was carried out in Scandinavia. There were not enough black patients to analyze. SOLVD was carried out in the U.S. under sponsorship of the National Institutes of Health. Since that study also compared enalapril to placebo I thought it should give us an opportunity to confirm our hypothesis. SOLVD was organized and supervised by Salim Yusuf, a cardiologist-epidemiologist who at the time was a program officer at the NIH. When he left the NIH to assume a cardiology post in Canada he maintained his access to the SOLVD data base. I called Salim to ask if he would do a quick analysis of the database to compare response to enalapril in the white and black population. He assured me that there was no difference but promised to re-analyze the data. He called me a couple days later to announce that he had re-checked the data and there was no difference.

I was not satisfied. Peter made me aware of a paper that was being prepared at the NIH re-analyzing the SOLVD database to show that black patients overall had poorer outcome than white patients. They had found what appeared to be a poorer response to enalapril in the black population but were pressured by the powers at the NIH not to emphasize that in the paper.

Megatrials

To understand the reluctance of these NIH investigators and of Salim Yusuf to find differences in therapeutic response requires understanding not only the sensitivity of the race issue but also the fundamental goal of clinical trialists.

Salim was a strong advocate for what is called "megatrials", a concept originated in England by a feisty clinical trialist named Richard Peto. Megatrials are carried out in very large and diverse populations of patients who are given a single drug or a placebo to determine the comparative effect on a simple non-controversial end-point, usually death. For example, if one wants to study whether one aspirin a day is beneficial, merely enter thousands of patients and give half of them aspirin and the other half a placebo. If it is a widely divergent population and there are fewer deaths in the aspirin group, one can extrapolate to the whole world population to estimate how many lives can be saved with aspirin.

What has always troubled me about the Peto-Yusuf philosophy is that it pre-supposes that differences in response among subpopulations are not important. Although megatrialists always go through the obligatory exercise of analyzing responses in obvious subpopulations—such as women vs. men, old people vs. young people, Asians or African-Americans vs. whites—the deck is always stacked against finding a difference. The subgroups are always too small to identify a statistically significant difference. The conclusion is always that no significant differences were observed in subpopulations.

That was Salim Yusuf's response when I asked him to explore the difference. Clinical trialists don't want to find a difference because it might invalidate their conclusion that the data from the megatrial can be applied to the world's population.

In interest of full disclosure, I must also reveal my own biased behavior. The V-HeFT racial re-analysis was concluded before Medco Research and I went to the FDA to plead for approval of BiDil for heart failure. We were seeking approval for the general population (albeit all male, an issue that never came up) studied in V-HeFT. I did not bring up the apparent racial difference in response because it would have weakened our argument for approval. If, in fact, BiDil was more effective in blacks, that would suggest it exhibited little benefit in whites. How could the FDA approve the drug under those circumstances? And since our analysis had not yet been published and was not known to Medco, I remained silent.

Unwilling to drop my effort at an unbiased re-analysis of SOLVD, I turned to one of the investigators at the NIH involved in the analysis of outcomes in blacks vs. whites. Derek Exner, who now is also a cardiologist in Canada, agreed to pursue the issue with a more powerful analytic tool.

When one tries to compare the response to enalapril vs. placebo in all the white patients and all the black patients in SOLVD, one is confronted with the striking differences in patient age, risk factors and severity of disease in the two populations, as well as a disproportion in the number of patients in the two racial subgroups. One way to overcome these problems is to match patients based on the characteristics that are likely to contribute to outcomes.

There were 800 black patients and 5719 white patients in the entire SOLVD study, which included two trials, one in patients with heart failure and another in patients with structural abnormalities of the left ventricle but no symptoms of heart failure. No other trial had ever studied such asymptomatic patients. The trick was to match up to four white patients with each black patient based on a list of characteristics that should eliminate gross predicted differences in outcome.

We identified 1196 white patients to match to our 800 black patients. Our hypothesis was confirmed. Enalapril reduced by 44% the risk of hospitalization for worsening heart failure in the white population—but not at all in the matched black population. We had verified one interpretation of our V-HeFT II re-analysis. ACE inhibitors are less effective in blacks than in whites who have structural damage to the heart and heart failure.

We were now ready to publish both our V-HeFT re-analysis and the re-analysis Derek Exner and I had performed on SOLVD. The medical world was going to be confronted with a new dilemma. Should all the advice about management of heart failure gleaned from large trials be modified for a racial subgroup that was under-represented in most of the trials? How would this controversial issue be viewed by my colleagues? The answer was not long in coming.

A hostile reception

Our first presentation of the data was met by an aggressive and hostile response, not only from clinical trialists whom I expected to disagree, but from many of my black cardiologist friends and colleagues. By suggesting that ACE inhibitors may not be as beneficial in blacks as in whites, I was threatening their effort to enhance use of effective drugs in blacks. Rather than seeing the data as raising a concern for their current treatment strategies in blacks, and as a stimulus for inclusion of more blacks in clinical trials, they viewed the data as conflicting with their efforts to get black patients treated comparably to white patients. They viewed disparate outcomes as a sign of disparate treatment. They did not want there to be a difference in response. They did not support any suggestion that blacks may be biologically different than whites—

certainly not our suggestion that there might be a genetic difference. I was in danger of being labeled a "racist".

NitroMed was fully aware of our racial re-analysis when it acquired the intellectual property for BiDil. The company was not concerned with the perception of some that the research was misguided. They felt that the data supported a unique benefit of BiDil in black patients, and since blacks have been reported to suffer disproportionately from heart failure and to have a poorer outcome with treatment, they felt that there was a remarkable opportunity to develop the drug for that specific population.

NitroMed made two decisions. It would apply for a patent utilizing the Carson/Cohn re-analyses of V-HeFT and V-HeFT II identifying a specific benefit of BiDil in black patients. And it would go back to the FDA with an NDA seeking approval of BiDil for heart failure in blacks.

The patent application was successful and the presentation to the FDA went surprisingly well. The agency was impressed with the racial data, especially because it was consistent with a well-accepted hypothesis. After much discussion, the FDA agreed that the retrospective re-analysis was so persuasive that it would issue an "approvable letter" to NitroMed stating that the drug combination could be approved if a follow-up study conducted specifically in a black population confirmed the benefit on outcome.

This was a watershed moment. The FDA not only did not criticize our distinction by race—an issue that would subsequently plague us—but suggested that it would approve a drug for a specific racial group. NitroMed agreed to support a new trial in blacks. It would be costly, so the company set out to raise the money. Sensitive to any potential backlash from the black community, the CEO, Michael Loberg, enlisted politically well-connected help. The Association of Black Cardiologists, an active group of mostly black physicians dedicated to enhancing care of this population, was enlisted the support of prominent black organizations. The Black Congressional Caucus was contacted, and I even went to Washington to meet with the caucus chairman, Congressman Townsend, to enlist his support. He was enthusiastically behind our effort and put a supporting document in the Congressional Record. Everything was in place. All we needed was a protocol, a study team, a thousand patients, analytical experts, and good luck. These elements were yet to come.

But the patent issue would come back to bite NitroMed. All drugs subjected to industry-sponsored clinical trials are protected by patents. No company wants to spend large sums of money studying a drug unless their intellectual property protects them from someone else making the drug and selling it. The patent protection on the use of ISDN/Hyd to treat heart failure had only a few years to go because it had been approved years before. That's why no large pharmaceutical companies were interested in developing the drug. NitroMed needed additional intellectual property to justify expenditure of the funds needed for a new trial. The new patent on use of BiDil to treat black patients with heart failure gave them the protection they needed. It was a sincere effort to improve treatment of heart failure in an underserved population, as well as a business decision, one that no responsible public company could proceed without. Yet some in the medical and lay community interpreted this as greediness. After effectiveness of the drug was proved in the trial, some claimed that the strategy to study and treat blacks was not based on science. That undeservedly negative view of NitroMed's motives, no different from that of any for-profit pharmaceutical company, would end up hurting the company and the NitroMed marketing strategy.

Had we proved that BiDil was more effective in blacks? Had we proved Salim Yusuf wrong when he concluded from his re-analysis of SOLVD that there was no racial difference in response to ACE inhibitors? Certainly not. As previously noted, post-hoc re-analysis of data can at best generate hypotheses, not proofs. A new study could never address any so-called racial difference in response to BiDil because it was going to be carried out in a single racial group. It will remain an unresolved issue until a large study is funded and conducted in a diverse population.

Should these data have changed the way we approached the treatment of heart failure? Should Sam Farber, a white man, have been treated with an ACE inhibitor when he developed heart failure, and should black patients be treated with BiDil? The answers are not simple.

The practice of medicine today has become what is now called "evidence-based." The evidence referred to usually comes from large-scale clinical trials demonstrating significant benefit in response to the therapy. The suggestion of a racial difference in drug response was based on retrospective analysis, a hypothesis-generating exercise, not a definitive prospective trial. Furthermore, racial designation was a very controversial topic.

Was race merely a crude approach to identifying genetic differences? Social scientists strongly criticized the idea, insisting that race is a social construct not a biological phenomenon. Genetic studies would be necessary to identify biological traits that may cluster in one population group versus another to account for differences in response. Geographic origin would be the most likely basis for distinction. Or did self-designated race uncover some environmental trait that influenced responsiveness? Were all these apparent differences merely a play of chance? Clearly the traditional concept of "evidence" was not adequately satisfied to justify guidelines to modify therapy based on self-designated race.

But doctors are free to make their own decisions when prescribing drugs. Back in the 1980s, after we had observed what appeared to be a remarkably favorable effect of isosorbide dinitrate and hydralazine, I began prescribing these drugs for my patients with heart failure. I thought the evidence was adequate to steer my drug management, even though the FDA had not agreed. When our early studies with ACE inhibitors demonstrated what I felt was a robust benefit, I began prescribing them to my patients, even though FDA approval was still years away. I assume many lives were saved by the use of effective drugs before the "evidence" satisfied regulatory bodies or guideline developers.

Similarly, after our re-analysis of V-HeFT, I began treating all black patients with isosorbide dinitrate and hydralazine. I was being pre-emptive, since the definitive study had not yet been done, but I was always eager to give my patients an advantage. That, after all, is part of the *art* of medicine, too often disregarded in these days of evidence-based guidelines.

CHAPTER XIII
African-American Heart Failure Trial
(A-HeFT)

Ten years passed between the completion in 1990 of V-HeFT II, the attempt to compare ISDN/Hyd with enalapril, and the initiation of the first study with the fixed-dose combination of the two drugs called BiDil. That delay wasn't based on science. It was related to the commercial interest of pharmaceutical companies who saw in heart failure the opportunity for new drugs.

BiDil was not a new drug that offered the prospect of big profits. Thanks to our studies with ISDN/Hyd and with ACE inhibitors, it was now clear that drugs could improve symptoms and slow progression of heart failure. Industry stood ready to respond to the challenge of new and better therapy. Those years were cluttered with clinical trials in heart failure, all designed to identify new or better drugs to treat this patient population.

The philosophy had changed. No longer were we seeking the best medication to treat heart failure—that is, enalapril vs. ISDN/Hyd. Now we were seeking the best drug combination. ACE inhibitors were now accepted as mandated therapy.

What could be added to the ACE inhibitor to further improve outcome? What kind of drugs was the industry trying to develop?

Pharmaceutical firms were exploring vasodilators, drugs that could improve heart function by lowering impedance, much as ISDN/Hyd did in V-HeFT. And they were seeking a drug that could stimulate the heart to beat more forcefully—hopefully a drug that could safely restore the heart's loss of contractile function. Although the industry pharmacologists now recognized the benefits on the circulation of relaxing the arteries, they could not escape the bias that the holy grail of therapy would be a drug that could enhance the heart's depressed contractile force.

V-HeFT III

In 1991, we initiated a study of another vasodilator as part of our "Vasodilator Heart Failure Trial (V-HeFT)" V.A. study philosophy. I took on this study because the pharmaceutical company offered support and I wanted to keep our outstanding team of V.A investigators intact. There was no funding for another ISDN/Hyd study. In this new trial, called V-HeFT III, we added the drug felodipine, a so-called calcium channel blocking agent, to existing background therapy with an ACE inhibitor. It was painful for me to design a study that excluded the use of ISDN/Hyd, but at the time we felt we could not add a potent vasodilator, felodpine, to another potent vasodilator regimen, ISDN/Hyd. And no drug company was interested in a comparative trial against ISDN-Hyd, which was not approved by the FDA. The only option was to study a drug vs. placebo in patients already treated with an ACE inhibitor.

Felodipine was marketed as Plendil for the treatment of hypertension. The marketing company was delighted with the prospect of an expanded approval for treatment of heart failure. They agreed to support a clinical trial.

After a study of 450 patients, we concluded that felodipine did not improve outcome in patients already treated with enalapril. Another study with a different calcium channel blocker, amlodipine (marketed as Norvasc), also failed to show benefit. So we now had further reason to question our initial vasodilator concept. Either the ACE inhibitor-induced benefit in these patients made an additional vasodilator unnecessary or vasodilation, which was certainly an action of these calcium channel blockers, was not the mechanism of the ISDN/Hyd benefit. Or maybe—and I resisted this thought—Bob Temple was right and ISDN/Hyd was no better than placebo.

Around that time I was approached regarding a new vasodilator drug being developed by Boots Pharmaceuticals. Two rather dashing young executives from Boots appeared in my office to brief me on the drug and seek my help in its development for heart failure. The male boss and female assistant were on a national tour meeting with thought leaders. Boots, a British firm, had an American branch in Louisiana where these two lived. From the experimental data they showed me, flosequinon appeared to have a dual effect as a vasodilator and a cardiac stimulant. Nothing could theoretically be more attractive for heart failure than a vasodilator that could improve LV emptying combined with an inotrope that could enhance contraction.

I was skeptical in getting involved for several reasons. I had become convinced that cardiac stimulants, though they might be useful short-term to improve depressed heart function, were likely to have long-term adverse effects on heart metabolism and heart rhythms. I much pre-ferred the improved function resulting from a vasodilator. Furthermore, this team from Boots seemed not up to the task of a complicated drug development program. I doubted if the expertise or funding would be able to meet the challenge. I did not offer my participation.

Boots went ahead and designed a study of flosequinon in chronic heart failure that was overseen by investigators from other institutions. Despite some improvement in heart function and symptoms, the drug led to an increase in mortality rate. Efforts to market it were dropped.

Another unique compound, vesnarinone, was developed by a Japa-nese company, Otsuka. It was purported to be a positive inotropic drug—that is, an agent that increases the force of heart muscle contraction. The sponsor had carried out a small clinical trial using two doses of the drug in an effort to identify the most effective dose, either 60 mg daily or 120 mg daily. Quite surprisingly, because they had not designed the trial to detect a survival benefit of the drug, the patients assigned to receive 60 mg vesnarinone had a highly significant 62% lower mortality than those assigned to receive placebo. Otsuka brought the trial results to the FDA to seek approval of the drug to reduce mortality in heart failure.

But there was a problem. The 120 mg dose had been withdrawn during the conduct of the study because of what appeared to be an increased mortality in that group. If 120 mg was harmful and 60 mg beneficial, what about 30 mg? How could the drug be approved for treatment when we knew so little about what we call the dose-response curve?

I was therefore skeptical of the data, and so was the FDA. The company agreed to perform a larger definitive trial. I knew Otsuka had the resources to pull it off. They asked me to chair the study and promised not to interfere with its conduct. I convinced them we would need to study two daily doses of the drug, 30 mg and 60 mg, in comparison to placebo in patients receiving all other approved therapy for heart failure.

From January 1995 to July 1996 we recruited in 189 medical centers in the U.S. and Canada a total of nearly 4000 patients who met the entrance criteria for the diagnosis of severe heart failure. When the study was terminated in July 1996 because the targeted number of total deaths had occurred, analysis revealed a dose-dependent increase in mortality (Figure XIII-1). That is, the 30 mg dose produced a modestly higher mortality than the placebo, and the 60 mg dose was associated with an even greater and statistically significant increase in mortality. Therefore, vesnarinone shortened life expectancy, not lengthened it. The earlier trial had been a fluke, a play of chance in a small population.

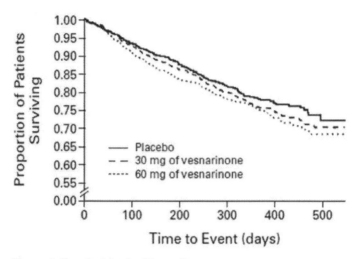

Figure 1. Survival in the Three Groups.

Figure XIII-1
Survival curves in patients with heart failure randomly assigned to receive, in addition to their standard therapy, vesnarinone 60 mg daily, vesnarinone 30 mg daily or place-bo. Note that survival was significantly reduced by incremental doses of vesnarinone.

So all this money spent by pharmaceutical companies – hundreds of millions of dollars for each study – had failed to identify a vasodilator or inotropic drug that could have a favorable effect on the dismal prognosis in patients with heart failure. Were ACE inhibitors and ISDN/Hyd destined to be the only effective treatment for heart failure?

A group of Swedish investigators became enamored with the use of beta blockers to treat heart failure. This was not a rational choice for drug therapy. It was not a vasodilator and it depressed cardiac function, not enhanced it. Indeed, it had long been taught that beta blockers were not to be used in patients with heart failure because they were likely to make the patient worse.

Beta blockers inhibit the sympathetic nervous system, which might make them attractive for use in a condition in which the sympathetic nervous system is activated. But they block the sympathetic activity to the heart, mediated by beta receptors, instead of blocking sympathetic activity to the blood vessels, which is mediated by alpha receptors. So the benefit observed by the Swedes was not easy to explain at the time. Perhaps, they thought, it was related to slowing the heart rate, which is a characteristic effect of beta blockers. And because of safety concerns, the investigators initiated the therapy at very low doses and gradually increased the dose over several weeks.

Clearly the beta blockers needed to be tested in large trials. Manufacturers of several of these compounds launched trials to test their drugs in patients already receiving ACE inhibitors. I played a leadership role in trials with one of these drugs, carvedilol or Coreg. When titrated properly from initially low doses, these beta blockers produced a remarkable reduction in mortality and reduction in the need for hospitalization. When we examined the effect of these drugs on cardiac structure it was apparent that they were profoundly inhibiting and even reversing the structural remodeling in the left ventricle.

So beta blockers became standard therapy for heart failure and were strongly advocated in all the practice guidelines developed late in the 1990s.

Angiotensin receptor blockers

A new class of drugs called angiotensin receptor blockers (ARBs) became available as an alternative way to inhibit the renin-angiotensin system. These drugs were becoming widely used as a substitute for ACE inhibitors to lower blood pressure in hypertensive patients. They act not to block the formation of angiotensin, like ACE inhibitors, but to block the activity of angiotensin by interfering with its effect on the blood vessels through interaction with the angiotensin receptor. The beauty of these new compounds was that they were not only effective in lowering blood pressure, but also remarkably free of side effects. As opposed to ACE inhibitors, which often lead to a cough and occasionally to severe allergic reactions, angiotensin receptor blockers (ARBs) are amazingly well tolerated.

Would ARBs work as well, or even better, than ACE inhibitors in patients with heart failure? How could we study the ARBs?

Since ACE inhibitors were now mandated therapy, we couldn't do a placebo-controlled trial without an ACE inhibitor. We could have designed a comparative trial in which half the patients were assigned to take the ARB and half the ACE inhibitor. But I've already expressed my discomfort with comparative trials. Even though the ARB and ACE inhibitor were both thought to work by inhibiting the renin-angiotensin system, their quite different modes of action made it possible that their effects could be quite different as well. Furthermore, we were no longer testing individual drugs. We were testing drug regimens.

I went to Novartis, the company that was selling valsartan, a potent ARB. They were enthusiastic about studying valsartan in patients with heart failure, but upper management was not pleased with my proposal to study it in patients already being treated with optimal therapy, including ACE inhibitors when tolerated. Furthermore, I was proposing a dose of valsartan much higher than they were advocating for the treatment of hypertension. And I proposed a twice-a-day dosing regimen rather than the once-daily strategy they were marketing for hypertension.

After gaining collaborative support from a group of Italian investigators led by Gianni Tognoni from Milan, and after additional meetings with Novartis, we gained their agreement with a protocol. Patients with moderate to severe heart failure, who were receiving all recommended and tolerated therapy but were still symptomatic, would be randomly assigned to receive either placebo or valsartan 160 mg twice daily.

The usual dose of valsartan recommended for hypertension at that time was 80 or 160 mg once daily. Our experience with the drug was that the absence of side effects would allow us to use higher and more effective doses without a problem. That turned out to be the case. The higher dose soon became standard for hypertension as well as heart failure.

Since some patients could not tolerate an ACE inhibitor, we knew that there would be an opportunity to study the effect of valsartan vs. placebo in the absence of an ACE inhibitor. But the major question we were addressing was whether adding valsartan to background therapy with an ACE inhibitor and often a beta blocker would result in better outcomes. We were seeking the optimal regimen for heart failure.

We named the study Val-HeFT, a clear extension of V-Heft but with valsartan as the vasodilator. Because I insisted that Novartis support collection of extensive ancillary mechanistic data as well as the clinical events that determine the outcome of a trial, this large international study (5010 patients, 16 countries) has generated dozens of publications providing new insights into heart failure. It also was able to demonstrate, much to Novartis' satisfaction, that valsartan exerted additional protective effects when added to an ACE inhibitor for heart failure. The FDA agreed and approved valsartan or Diovan as therapy for heart failure.

BiDil

BiDil was different. It was a nitric oxide donor, not a hormone inhibitor. If nitric oxide was important in inhibiting structural remodeling, and if it was deficient in patients with heart failure, then BiDil might be effective even in patients whose deleterious hormone systems were already blocked with standard therapy. If our post-hoc analysis of V-HeFT was correct, then black patients might exhibit on average a greater deficiency of nitric oxide than white patients and might reasonably be expected to respond better to BiDil. The previous evidence of nitric oxide deficiency in blacks supported this hypothesis.

So A-HeFT was designed as a trial of BiDil, but was actually planned to be a test of the nitric oxide hypothesis. Such a mechanistic approach to clinical trial design is not viewed favorably by most of the clinical trial community. Trialists scoff at the idea that they are testing a mechanistic hypothesis. They test specific therapies, they claim, and mechanisms can never be inferred from a large clinical trial. We know too little about human disease, they claim, to ever be certain about mechanisms. All we can know, they insist, is whether a treatment has had a favorable overall effect.

I cling to the mechanistic approach. Medical research is not like baseball games, football games or elections, when winning is everything and losing is nothing. I counsel young investigators never to undertake a study when the only useful outcome is the positive result sought. If a single drug fails, it may be of little import, but if a study can exclude a mechanism of disease, it can have great value. All studies, then, should be designed so that a negative result may be as important as a positive result.

In A-HeFT we would explore the nitric oxide hypothesis with the only drug purported to enhance its production, the combination of isosorbide dinitrate and hydralazine now known as BiDil.

We selected an acronym for the study. We had done V-HeFT for the vasodilator heart failure trials. We had just finished Val-HeFT for the valsartan (an angiotensin receptor blocker) heart failure trial, and I was involved on the steering committee for SCD-HeFT, the sudden cardiac death heart failure trial. I thought we needed a new –HeFT study title. Since it was to be performed in a single racial group, it needed to reflect that population. The choices were B-HeFT for black heart failure trial or A-HeFT for African-American heart failure trial. I could get no unanimity on whether black or African-American was the preferred terminology. African-American seemed to me the more scholarly term, but it was pointed out that there are many white Africans living in America who would not be eligible for the study. In our previous publication on racial distinctions published in the *New England Journal of Medicine,* the editors had dutifully replaced all of our designations of African Americans with the term "black". I conferred with many of my black African-American colleagues and got shrugs of indifference. We decided to go with A-HeFT.

Designing the study

A first order of business was to identify a chairman of the study to oversee its conduct. I could not take that on because I was conflicted by my contract with NitroMed. I could not be an independent investigator because I stood to gain from a successful trial. I could serve only as a company representative on the study. Furthermore, I felt we needed a black cardiologist to bring credibility to the study design. That would help in recruiting investigators to participate as well as to report the results of the study to colleagues. My search ended quickly with a gift from heaven: Anne Taylor.

Anne appeared in my office as a potential candidate for a position in the medical school. Anne was an experienced academic cardiologist who was on the faculty at Case Western Reserve in Cleveland where she had interacted with our Chairman of Medicine, Jonathan Ravdin, who had been a professor in Cleveland prior to his arrival in Minneapolis. Jonathan was trying to recruit her to join the cardiology faculty and to serve also as an associate dean in the medical school. Anne was not only an experienced clinician and investigator, but she was also black and an active member of the Association of Black Cardiologists (ABC). I discussed the proposed study with her and suspect that her acceptance of the university position was related to the opportunity to become chair of the trial. It was a perfect fit.

The study would address a spectrum of interests: scientific, clinical and business. The study team would encompass them all: My dedication was to the whole spectrum, but the science took precedence and my financial interest couldn't be disregarded. Anne was excited by the science and the opportunity to improve management of heart failure in blacks. NitroMed's commitment was to raise the company's net worth and stock price while providing a drug that could enhance the well-being and life expectancy of black patients. It was a potential win-win for all.

The protocol was a bit more complicated. NitroMed had limited funds available for the study so we needed to keep the population modest in size. Furthermore, no one had previously tried to recruit an exclusively black population of patients with heart failure and I was concerned it might be difficult. We had to make certain that our endpoint was sensitive enough to pick up a drug-induced difference in the available patient population. In the 4000+ patient Val-HeFT study we had elected to use a combined primary outcome—mortality plus hospitalization for worsening heart failure—to enhance the power of demonstrating a benefit of valsartan.

The power of a trial is related to the number of target events that occur during the follow-up period. The number of events, of course, depends on what you decide to count and how long you follow the patients. If you select death as the end-point, your study must continue until enough patients have died to identify a benefit of the experimental treatment over the placebo group. This is usually accomplished by planning to follow the patients until a specific number of deaths have occurred, that number having been calculated by the biostatisticians to provide adequate power to test the hypothesis that the treatment will be effective.

In Val-HeFT we were concerned that deaths alone would not give us adequate power so we decided to add hospitalizations for worsening heart failure as an additional primary end-point. Therefore, what we were studying is whether treatment with valsartan would reduce the risk of the patient either dying or requiring hospital admission for worsening heart failure. It's a bit complicated to use a dual primary end-point such as this because the end-points are in a way "competitive". If the patient dies, he or she cannot subsequently be hospitalized, but if the patient is hospitalized, he or she can subsequently die. Thus the time to death and the time to the primary event may be strikingly different.

Outcomes

The combined end-point in Val-HeFT was improved by valsartan compared to placebo when the drugs were added to all other background medication. But we could demonstrate no significant benefit on mortality alone (Figure XIII-2), so we were fortunate to have chosen a combined end-point.

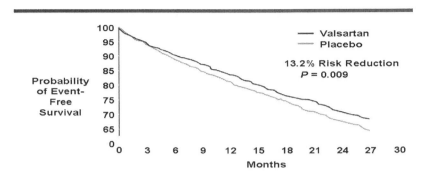

Cohn JN et al. *N Engl J Med*. 2001;345:1667-1675.

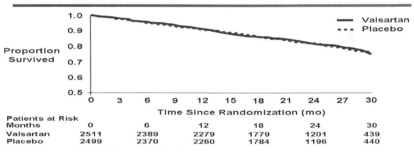

*P value (log-rank): 0.801; hazard ratio (Cox model): 1.017.
Cohn JN et al. *N Engl J Med*. 2001;345:1667-1675.

Figure XIII-2

Graphs displaying event-free survival (death or hospitalization for heart failure) in the two treatment arms (first graph) and survival alone (second graph). Valsartan significantly improved the combined end-point but did not affect mortality. The patients were well-treated with all other therapy known to affect survival.

It must be kept in mind that a clinical trial succeeds or fails depending on its achievement of the primary end-point goal. Biostatistical practice mandates that if the trial fails to achieve its primary end-point, it is a negative trial regardless of what other information can be gleaned from post-study analysis of other data. Had we chosen mortality as the end-point, the benefit on hospitalization for heart failure would have fallen into the category of an "interesting hypothesis". Since we used the combined end-point, the results were deemed to be statistically defensible and the FDA subsequently approved valsartan for the management of heart failure.

In planning A-HeFT, we needed to choose a primary end-point that was likely to demonstrate the benefit of BiDil in a smaller population that we would be able to fund and recruit. Although our re-analysis of V-HeFT had revealed a 47% mortality reduction in the black population, I didn't believe A-HeFT could come close to that magnitude of benefit. This had been a retrospective analysis of a small subset of the V-HeFT data and unlikely to be replicable, I thought. Furthermore, V-HeFT was performed in patients on no background therapy whereas we would now be doing a study in patients receiving multiple drugs that had been shown to reduce mortality. Death could not be the primary end-point, and I thought even death plus heart failure hospitalization might not generate enough events for statistical significance.

Choosing a composite end-point was a challenge. I had always been troubled by trial end-points that depend on morbid events. Only a minority of patients in any study experience a morbid event such as death or heart failure hospitalization during the limited follow-up period of the study. That means that most of the patients in the trial do not contribute to the end-point. They are basically "noise" in the study, data that do not influence the final result. Is there not a way, I reasoned, to include everyone in the end-point assessment? Since everyone takes a study drug, wouldn't it be better to assess everyone's response, not just those who have an event?

The easiest way, I thought, would be to give everyone a score for their health at the end of the study. Morbid events would certainly be an important contributor to the score, but we also needed a way to assess everyone's quality of life as a more sensitive guide to a favorable therapeutic response. This is where the Minnesota Living with Heart Failure Questionnaire became critical.

Quality of life

In the early 1980s I hired Tom Rector, a young pharmacist-biostatistician, to work in our research program to help with protocol design and data analysis. As one of his early tasks, I assigned him to come up with a questionnaire that heart failure patients could fill out to characterize the adverse effects of heart failure on their quality of life. Nothing like that had been developed and I thought it would be a useful way to track patients' response to treatment.

Tom approached the assignment in a scholarly way. He developed test questionnaires that he administered to patients with heart failure to find out what aspect of their lives seemed to be most affected by their disease. He gradually honed it down to 21 questions that assessed both physical limitations imposed by heart failure and emotional or psychological effects of their impaired performance and health care requirements. The 21 questions are displayed in Figure XIII-3.

LIVING WITH HEART FAILURE QUESTIONNAIRE

These questions concern how your heart failure (heart condition) has prevented you from living as you wanted during the last month. The items listed below describe different ways some people are affected. If you are sure an item does not apply to you or is not related to your heart failure then circle 0 (No) and go on to the next item. If an item does apply to you, then circle the number rating how much it prevented you from living as you wanted. Remember to think about ONLY THE LAST MONTH.

Did your heart failure prevent you from living as you wanted during the last month by:	No	Very little				Very much
1. Causing swelling in your ankles, legs, etc?	0	1	2	3	4	5
2. Making you sit or lie down to rest during the day?	0	1	2	3	4	5
3. Making your walking about or climbing stairs difficult?	0	1	2	3	4	5
4. Making your working around the house or yard difficult?	0	1	2	3	4	5
5. Making your going places away from home difficult?	0	1	2	3	4	5
6. Making your sleeping well at night difficult?	0	1	2	3	4	5
7. Making your relating to or doing things with your friends or family difficult?	0	1	2	3	4	5
8. Making your working to earn a living difficult?	0	1	2	3	4	5
9. Making your recreational pastimes, sports or hobbies difficult?	0	1	2	3	4	5
10. Making your sexual activities difficult?	0	1	2	3	4	5
11. Making you eat less of the foods you like?	0	1	2	3	4	5
12. Making you short of breath?	0	1	2	3	4	5
13. Making you tired, fatigued, or low on energy?	0	1	2	3	4	5
14. Making you stay in a hospital?	0	1	2	3	4	5
15. Costing you money for medical care?	0	1	2	3	4	5
16. Giving you side effects from medications?	0	1	2	3	4	5
17. Making you feel you are a burden to your family or friends?	0	1	2	3	4	5
18. Making you feel a loss of self-control in your life?	0	1	2	3	4	5
19. Making you worry?	0	1	2	3	4	5
20. Making it difficult for you to concentrate or remember things?	0	1	2	3	4	5
21. Making you feel depressed?	0	1	2	3	4	5

Copyright University of Minnesota, 1986.

Figure XIII-3

The 21 questions in the Minnesota Living with Heart Failure Questionnaire. A total score is obtained from the sum of each score.

The unique aspect of this so-called quality of life assessment, however, was that the score reported by the patient was not so much dependent on their symptoms as on how much the disability, whatever it was, affected their ability to live life as they wanted to. It wasn't a symptom score but a quality of life score. For instance, if their ankles were swollen from heart failure, it was only important if the swelling in some way adversely affected their life style or their perception of health.

Since its introduction, the Minnesota Living with Heart Failure Questionnaire (MLHFQ) has been widely used internationally to quantify the effect of therapy in multiple trials and track benefits in clinical practice. It was copyrighted by the University of Minnesota so its use has required a license and a modest fee, which is paid to the University of Minnesota, some of which is steered to Tom and me as inventors. The use has been so widespread that I understand our Office of Patents and Technology has collected more money on this little questionnaire than on most of the other inventions developed in recent years by the University. Although it had been used frequently in clinical trials in order to document beneficial effects in a patient, it had not been used as a primary end-point of a study. I thought that this was the opportunity.

How could we use it in combination with morbid events such as death and hospitalization for heart failure? A scoring system needed to be devised. Death is certainly the worst outcome for a patient, so I assigned a score of -3 for any patient who died during the follow-up period, which we arbitrarily truncated at 18 months. Being hospitalized for heart failure, as opposed to other causes that we were not treating, is certainly adverse, but not as bad as death. I assigned it a score of -1.

Our previous experience with the MLHFQ had convinced me that a change in score of 10 units or more was always accompanied by objective measures of clinical change, such as improved or worsening exercise tolerance on a stress test. Such a change in MHLHFQ score, favorable or unfavorable, I thought deserved a score of 2. Changes between 5 and 10 were often more subtle, so I assigned them a score of 1. Changes less than 5 were not counted because they could represent normal variation of scoring. We also had to set a specific time after randomization to establish the change in MLHFQ. It had to be a time long enough to observe the effects of treatment but short enough for almost all patients to reach the point and be counted. I decided on six months.

So the score change at the end of the trial could go from +2 for a patient whose MLHFQ score improved by 10 units at six months and neither died nor was hospitalized during the 18-month follow-up, to -6 for a patient who had a decline in MLHFQ at six months, was hospitalized and subsequently died within 18 months. Everyone would now have a score, even if it was zero. Every patient in the trial would contribute to the primary end-point. It was a striking departure from previous cardiovascular disease trial designs.

Who is eligible for the study?

We then had to decide who should be included in the study. First of all, participants had to identify themselves as African American or black. That was their decision, not ours. We wanted men and women, particularly women because there were no prior data on treatment of women with the drug combination now called BiDil. We wanted them to be very symptomatic with their heart failure so that we could more easily detect improvement, and also because more severely symptomatic patients have a higher risk of hospitalization and death, which were important contributors to our primary end-point.

The standard way to assess severity of heart failure is with a ranking system developed years ago by the New York Heart Association. This classification identifies patients with symptoms even at rest as Class IV, those with symptoms on normal daily activity as Class III, those with symptoms only with unusual activity as Class II, and those without symptoms as Class I. We decided to confine the study to Class III and IV, although we fully recognized the subjective nature of this classification system.

The severity of structural change in the left ventricle—the pumping chamber of the heart—correlates surprisingly poorly with the severity of symptoms, but enlargement of the heart is a powerful predictor of premature death. We clearly wanted patients whose hearts had enlarged and whose ejection fraction, as defined in Chapter 9, was reduced. We established eligibility criteria based on an ultrasound (echocardiography) measurement of left ventricular structure and function.

We also needed to establish a dosing regimen. V-HeFT had used a target dose of 40 mg isosorbide dinitrate and 75 mg hydralazine four times daily. When we examined pill usage, however, we found that most patients usually took it only three times daily. So to simplify the regimen we decided to prescribe it three times a day. Since the BiDil tablet was formulated with 20 mg isosorbide dinitrate and 37.5 mg hydralazine we would need to start everyone on one pill three times a day and increase it, if tolerated, to two tablets three times daily. Half the patients would receive the BiDil tablets and half would receive matching placebo tablets.

When one plans a pivotal study for FDA approval, as this study was, the protocol must be reviewed with the agency so that the sponsor can be assured that a positive result will lead to drug approval. We went again to the FDA to present our plan for a trial designed to respond to their "approvable" letter with the confirmatory study they had requested. I had some trepidation about our scoring system. It was an entirely new end-point that had never been validated. The FDA could have insisted that we confine ourselves to events, such as death and hospitalization, which other studies had done. But the agency agreed that quality of life was a clinically meaningful assessment and the MLHFQ had been validated in previous trials. They recognized that our scoring system was arbitrary and then made an unsurprising statement: *You can use any composite scoring system you want as your primary endpoint, but we will look individually at the components of that end-point to be certain all of the important clinical events are going in the right direction.* In other words, the FDA was saying that we could not bury deaths and hospitalization in a composite score. They would tease them out. We could meet our primary goal with the scoring system, but if deaths or hospitalizations go in the wrong direction we won't get approval.

The sample size dilemma

The problem of sample size had to be resolved. When designing a pure "event" trial it is customary to recruit a pre-specified number of patients and then follow them until the number of events by which you have powered the study have occurred. The follow-up time is therefore not prescribed. In a study with the A-HeFT design, however, follow-up time is prescribed and the variable is then the number of patients needed to be entered into the trial. Based on retrospective application of our A-HeFT scoring system to our old V-HeFT data, our biostatisticians had estimated that a population of 800 patients might give us adequate power to detect the benefit of BiDil. But in the absence of experience with this scoring system we knew the estimate was risky and might result in too small a study group to adequately test the hypothesis.

Here is where the FDA gave us a surprising hand. It took the unusual step of allowing our independent data monitoring committee to examine the data partway through the study to recalculate, based on the early data, how many patients would be needed to test the hypothesis. The initial estimate of 400 patients per treatment group, or 800 patients altogether, was increased at that time to 1100 patients or 550 assigned to each treatment.

All trials performed by small companies are carried out with the help of a clinical research organization (CRO). These are for-profit organizations that recruit study centers and investigators for the sponsor, train study personnel, develop case report forms on which all clinical data are recorded, monitor the progress of the study, collect all the data forms, and often carry out statistical analysis of the results. Their work is critical to the success of the study and their budget is one of the biggest expenses of a study.

. Investigators often form a love-hate relationship with CROs. The CRO usually wants to run things, whereas the chairman of the study and the study medical leaders often feel that they should be in charge. The CRO personnel in the field may have little insight into the disease being studied so their advice to study sites often may be misleading. The confrontation between investigators and CRO can sometimes interfere with the conduct of a study.

Recruitment

With A-HeFT, a number of missteps almost destroyed the study in its initial phases. Recruitment of sites to perform the study is a critical first step. In an effort to identify centers with black patients—and because of the involvement of the Association of Black Cardiologists (ABC)—the CRO went to black physicians with clinical trial experience. Unfortunately, most of that experience was in hypertension trials, often in primary care practice. It turned out that many of those physicians did not see patients with heart failure, certainly not the kind of advanced heart failure we were studying, and many of them had little experience or expertise in treating heart failure. Susan Ziesche was plagued with data from patients with improper diagnoses, improper background therapy and poorly performed baseline tests.

Some of the sites chosen to participate by the CRO were weird. One investigator, who none of us knew, submitted several data forms that suggested patients inappropriately selected for the study. A site visit was planned to check on the center. The doctor arranged to meet the site visitors at a convenience store rather than at his office. The site visitors never saw an office and were left with the impression that he did not have an office or that at least it was not suitable for visitors. It was clear that he was not experienced in heart failure and did not have the facility to manage it. He was promptly dismissed from the study and any data on his patients were eliminated. A mid-course correction led to recruitment of more appropriate centers and cardiologists who knew how to treat heart failure.

The first patient was randomized on June 12, 2001, but recruitment was slow. Efforts were made to market the study in black neighborhoods, black churches and even barber shops. The ABC was valuable in getting the message out to black doctors. Eventually, more than 160 centers were recruited to screen patients for participation in the study. We had hoped to complete entering new patients into the trial in less than three years. Although recruitment remained slower than anticipated, as it has been in every study I have been involved in, it appeared that we were on track to reach our goal of 1100 patients.

The DSMB

The Data Safety and Monitoring Board DSMB met at 6-month intervals as outlined in its charter. At a meeting in April 2004, however, they requested an early update for a meeting in three months. This sort of request always means that the committee is observing something that may require some change in the protocol, or even premature termination of the trial. No committee likes to terminate a trial prematurely. The statistical power of a study and all the secondary endpoints and mechanistic data being collected benefit from a full database of the prescribed number of patients and their follow-up.

There are three possible reasons to recommend early termination. One is for unanticipated adverse effects of the study drug that make it unethical to continue administering it to patients. The DSMB is the protector of the patients who have agreed to participate. When they conclude from their review of the data that patients are being harmed they are ethically responsible to recommend termination. This seemed highly unlikely to us based on the long history of use of these drugs and our previous experience.

A second reason is "futility". Not all DSMBs are empowered to consider "futility", but it is a useful strategy when evaluating a new intervention that is not currently available for clinical use. If the study is powered to identify, for example, a 25% reduction in mortality from the intervention, and after 75% of the patients have been recruited there is absolutely no trend for a benefit, the committee may elect to project possible outcomes when all the patients are recruited. If it is apparent that there is no way additional data will change the conclusion of "no effect", it might be appropriate to consider terminating the trial to protect new patients from participating in a doomed trial and reduce further expenditures on a useless therapy. This could not have been the case in this study. The primary end-point on which we had powered the study was a score which the DSMB was not actually monitoring. Morbid events and deaths, which it was monitoring, could not lead to a conclusion of "futility" since the score would ultimately determine the outcome.

The third reason is the most exciting. If the observed benefit of a therapy is far greater than was predicted, then the study might not need to continue until its planned completion to document that the treatment is effective. The statistical tests for early termination are particularly stringent. P-values of 0.05 or 0.01 are not adequate because under these circumstances the committee does not want to be wrong even once in a hundred times. The treatment effect must be so dramatic that there can be *no doubt*. In fact, the committee is essentially saying to the doctors and patients that this treatment is so effective that all patients should be taking it, not just the half assigned to that therapy. The DSMB is protecting the placebo group from continued treatment without the effective drug. Since the committee was monitoring mortality, it would need to have observed so many fewer deaths in the treatment group that it could not justify continuing the study. Although we dared not to speculate about the committee's request for an early re-review of the data, it seemed to us that this third possibility was the most likely.

Then came July 17, 2004. I was on the tennis court on that Saturday when Anne Taylor called my cell phone. The DSMB had recommended stopping the study for lack of safety in the placebo group. At that time, 54 patients had died in the placebo group and only 32 in the BiDil group. When the time-dependent survival curves were examined, this represented a 43% reduction in mortality, an effect that could have happened by chance less than once in well over 100 times. When viewed in light of the similar benefit observed in V-HeFT, the committee felt that it was no longer ethical to randomize patients to receive placebo. Equipoise had been shattered.

I served two aces and went home to celebrate. Or at least that's how I remember it.

NitroMed takes action

A recommendation by a DSMB is only that. The DSMB reported directly to the study sponsor, NitroMed, who controlled the study's conduct. NitroMed agreed with the recommendation and pledged to notify all centers to discontinue the study as of Monday, July 19th. Furthermore, as a public company, NitroMed was required to issue a press release simultaneous with notification of the individual centers because of the material nature of the decision and its potential impact on its stock price. Any purchase of shares prior to public disclosure was sure to raise the interest of federal authorities. Thankfully, the stock price of NitroMed started to soar only after public disclosure.

Stopping a study is at least as complicated as starting one, especially when it is stopped prematurely for a favorable effect. All patients must be scheduled to come back so they can be notified of the results. That takes days or weeks, depending on schedules, during which study medication is continued. Patients immediately want to know whether they were taking BiDil or placebo, but the code cannot be broken until all the report forms from all the patients have been received and verified. That process is called "locking the data base". If the code were broken before that had taken place, potential bias could enter into the process.

What does one do in the meantime? Based on the DSMB's justification for stopping the study—which was that *not* taking the drug was *unsafe*—all patients should now receive the active drug BiDil. Half of them were already receiving the drug and should continue it, but the other half were on placebo and should be given BiDil. *But we didn't know which half.* Furthermore, BiDil was an experimental drug not approved for clinical use. We needed a "Compassionate Use" protocol approved by each of the institution's review boards to even administer this medication now that the A-HeFT study was terminated. Fortunately, the process of approving a compassionate use protocol had already been started so that the drug was ready to be offered to the patients.

Developing a strategy for transitioning patients from blinded drug therapy to known BiDil required considerable ingenuity. Everyone had to be started on a low dose and the dose gradually increased. Those already taking BiDil would be unnecessarily inconvenienced, but the patients on placebo would require gradual escalation of the dose as tolerated.

We also had to deal with the likelihood that there would be a landslide of requests from doctors and patients to have access to BiDil even if they were not enrolled in A-HeFT. The magnitude of the benefit, we thought, would lead to a storm of requests. We decided that "compassionate use" would be confined to the A-HeFT population and not to the heart failure population of black people at large because of the complexity and cost of providing drug to a large population. NitroMed instead committed itself to efforts to facilitate "data lock", data analysis, and submission to the FDA for prompt approval.

The press release from NitroMed generated widespread media attention. *The Wall Street Journal* and *The New York Times* ran prominent stories reporting the startling results of the study and speculating about FDA approval of a drug for a specific racial group. Some of the media presented opinions challenging the performance of a study specifically in blacks. We had anticipated some of the critical responses, but the intensity of hostility in some of the opinion pieces surprised us. We were particularly chagrined that the most vehement protests came from individuals in the black community who would be the beneficiaries of the new therapy.

The responsibility of the investigators was to plan presentation and publication of the results as soon as possible. Anne and I conferred about the process. Final data analysis could not be initiated until "data lock". That left a relatively short time to put together a presentation for the meeting of the American Heart Association in November. I presented the historical background, including V-HeFT, and Anne presented the dramatic results of A-HeFT (Figure XIII-4).

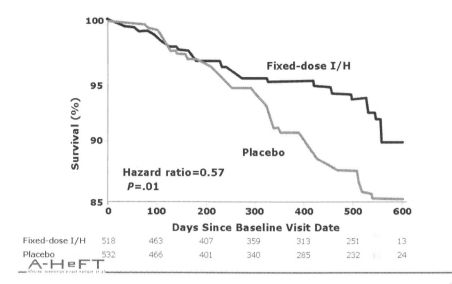

Figure XXX-4

Survival curves in African American black patients treated with BiDil (Fixed-dose I/H) or placebo. The mortality rate was reduced by 43%.

The media again featured the results. The *New York Times* reported the data as "vindicating" me (I may have suggested that word) after more than 20 years of waiting.

As we subsequently analyzed the other data from A-HeFT, the magnitude and mechanism of the benefit above and beyond mortality reduction became even more apparent. Hospitalizations for heart failure were strikingly reduced, quality of life was remarkably improved, the left ventricle became smaller and the ejection fraction rose in the BiDil treated patients compared to the placebo group. Nitric oxide enhancement had surpassed our most optimistic predictions. And its effect was superimposed on all the background therapy previously shown to be life-saving.

The FDA meets again

FDA approval was the only remaining obstacle. We had hoped they might approve the drug without a formal meeting, because they had already issued a "letter of approval" dependent only on successful completion of A-HeFT. But this would be a new approved treatment for heart failure and in a specific subgroup of the population.

The agency felt it needed a committee hearing. We were scheduled to present the data. The only issue, really, was whether the FDA would stick to its willingness to approve a drug for a racial category. The battle lines in the community were growing. Michael Loberg was concerned that a broader approval would allow generic drug companies to compete in the marketplace because the patent on overall use had a short life. It was the patent on use in black patients that gave the company long-term security.

As it turned out the committee meeting went smoothly, despite several comments during the open public hearing by antagonists to the use of racial profiling. We presented the data that were essentially non-controversial. The agency never expressed concern about the precedent for approving a drug for a single racial group. The drug was approved for black patients with heart failure and NitroMed's main agenda was training a sales force and preparing for marketing. All the hurdles had been scaled. I was pleased that my drug invention and my long-term commitment to a mechanistic approach to treatment would finally benefit a large population of sick people. Anne was delighted that her effort in chairing the study would be rewarded by improved health care for black patients. NitroMed was prepared to watch their profits grow while basking in the limelight of an important contribution to health care.

We were all grossly over-optimistic.

CHAPTER XIV
Marketing a Drug

I thought that the magnitude of benefit of BiDil in the black population combined with the notoriety of press coverage of the study and the FDA deliberations would propel prescriptions for the drug. Of course, a sales force is necessary, but this drug should sell itself, I thought.

NitroMed apparently felt the same way. They projected, to the pleasure of their stockholders, that sales would reach more than $200 million a year. In his enthusiasm, Mike Loberg made what I thought was a critical error. I had always anticipated that the BiDil drug combination would sell at a price somewhere between the cost of the generic components and the other patent-protected drugs which had been shown to be effective for heart failure.

The best example was Coreg, the beta blocker that had gained approval by the FDA at the same time that they had rejected BiDil when it was owned by Medco Research. After a slow marketing start Coreg had become a billion dollar drug for heart failure. Mike thought that since the BiDil data were even more dramatic than Coreg data, BiDil should be priced accordingly. He underestimated the sales impact of a gigantic marketing budget by GlaxoSmithKline, the owner of Coreg, and the sensitivity of the population for whom BiDil was intended. I pleaded with Mike to reduce the proposed price, but he insisted it would be offset by a generous program of free drug to those in need. Such programs, like many hand-outs, seldom work in practice.

The launch of BiDil

Big pharmaceutical companies launch new products with high profile sales events. NitroMed, despite its modest size, was not to be outdone. A gala event in Miami gathered together all the new sales agents that NitroMed had hired along with key investigators and NitroMed executives. It was a celebration that featured black entertainers and black motivational speakers. The music was loud. The sales force was enthused. Since they work on commission, sales reps could envision their incomes rising briskly. Like the housing market bubble, the mood was soon to be deflated.

It's hard to explain why things went badly. The sales force was small, inexperienced and had no idea how to identify doctors who saw black patients with heart failure. They were distributed across the country in population centers, but there weren't enough reps in any city to cover very many doctors. A rising drumbeat of negative views was being heard. The high price of the drug was interpreted as an attempt by NitroMed to cash in on the backs of poor black people, even though insurance coverage for the drug was progressively expanding. The mere fact that the drug was being marketed for blacks was turned against the company with accusations that NitroMed did not want to study whites because of its patent protection for blacks, an issue that we have already addressed extensively.

Another possible explanation for sluggish sales was that physicians were prescribing the cheaper generic drugs in an effort to replicate the effects of the expensive BiDil. But the company was watching the sales of isosorbide dinitrate and hydralazine. A small bump-up in the sales of these generic drugs probably represented prescriptions for heart failure, but the sales represented only a small additional use.

The public response

The academic community joined in. A high-profile symposium was organized by the University of Minnesota Law School to explore use of ethnicity in medical research. It became clear that the agenda was to address the BiDil issue. Nationally recognized social scientists and anthropologists criticized the whole concept of race as a biologically distinguishable feature. One highly regarded black professor of law at a prestigious Midwestern university was highly incensed by the introduction of self-identified race into therapeutic decision-making. She insisted that she would refuse to be taken care of by any doctor who based any decision on her being black. She even said she would rather die of heart failure than take a drug that had been specifically developed for black people with heart failure. Unfortunately, such critics are preoccupied with avoiding distinction by race, no matter how it is defined. They fail to appreciate the difference between *laws of the land*, which should treat everyone as equal, and *laws of nature*, which do not.

A young lawyer-turned-bioethicist, Jonathan Kahn, began publishing a series of articles (all basically the same) accusing NitroMed (and, by inference, me and my colleagues) of unethical practice in studying black people for financial gain. He recently published a book based on these commentaries, *Race in a Bottle*, which was assessed in a largely negative review in the *New York Times Science* section on December 25, 2012. The *Science Times* published my letter expressing disagreement with the book a week later.

I participated in radio call-in shows where some listeners expressed admiration for our work but others were hostile about the whole idea that black patients should be differentiated from white patients. We had apparently crossed a dangerous line. It was fine to identify blacks as a socially-deprived minority, but not to even suggest that there might be a biological difference.

This oppositional hyperbole was not questioning individual variability, but rather the use of racial characteristics—even if self-identified—as the defining feature. Clearly, it is not race itself but rather some genetic and possibly environmental characteristics of that population that influences biology.

We collected bloods on most of the patients in A-HeFT and got their permission to study DNA. There were certainly differences in this black

population in the frequency of certain genetic markers compared to previously studied white populations. Did those differences account for the
favorable response to BiDil? There was no way to tell. None of the
differences could be attributed to a single gene variation or any single
marker. Much as we would like to be able to characterize the responsiveness trait more specifically, such identifiers do not currently exist
and are unlikely to become available in the near future. Geographic origin or ethnicity is the only characteristic currently available. To deny the
drug's use because of racial sensitivity reduces the ability of physicians
to make therapeutic decisions that can improve the precision of disease
management.

NitroMed gives up

As sales languished at about $10 million per year, hardly enough
to support NitroMed's modest marketing effort, the company began to
curtail marketing. It became clear, if prior experience had not been an
adequate teacher, that success in marketing requires deep financial resources and an aggressive campaign strategy. NitroMed had neither of
these. The data were there. The patients were there. The need was there.
But black patients remained untreated with BiDil. The message apparently was not out, or at least had not been heard and turned into action.

Physicians are stubborn. They do not easily change what they do.
That's why pharmaceutical companies have begun marketing more and
more to the public to get consumers to push doctors for prescriptions.
The success of TV ads for restless leg syndrome, a medical condition
of dubious reality, and for drugs such as Vytorin or Zetia, whose effectiveness has now been questioned, provides insight into how financial
resources—not necessarily science—drive sales. Public advertising is a
very expensive marketing strategy.

NitroMed was in no position to fund such an effort. In fact, NitroMed's stock price was falling from its high near 30 after the excitement of BiDil had peaked to less than a dollar. Mike Loberg was removed as CEO by the Board of Directors. Manuel Worcel moved on to

other ventures. Most of the team that had worked to develop BiDil left the company. All research activity was discontinued. The sales force was terminated. Indeed, after the sales force left, the sales of BiDil did not change, thus confirming their ineffectiveness. In 2009, the company was sold for a tiny fraction of its market capitalization at the peak of the BiDil mania.

The rise and fall of NitroMed serves as a lesson in business schools around the country. Was BiDil's failure to penetrate the marketplace an insurmountable obstacle erected by racial sensitivity, or did it reflect a failed strategy by the vender? Does it suggest that only big pharma, with deep pockets of cash, can successfully market a new drug? Apparently drugs need to be marketed aggressively to get physicians to write prescriptions. Scientific articles in the *New England Journal of Medicine* and news reports in *The New York Times* and *The Wall Street Journal* are not adequate to sell drugs.

What is the future of BiDil? The entity that bought the company, a holding company called Deerfield Associates, spent the first year reviewing its options to make the product successful. The company offered to sell BiDil to several small companies while considering the mounting of a new marketing effort itself. Eventually, BiDil was sold to Arbor Pharmaceuticals, a specialty pharmaceutical company based in Atlanta that sells drugs in the cardiovascular and pediatric market place. Arbor claims to be planning an expanded marketing effort.

Meanwhile, renewed interest in nitric oxide enhancement in the cardiology community has sparked the design of new studies to test the effectiveness of BiDil in non-black patients with heart failure, and possibly in other cardiovascular diseases that may benefit from nitric oxide enhancement. The National Institutes of Health has been approached about supporting a large-scale outcomes trial that may at last resolve the question as to whether BiDil works for all patients or only those of African American descent. Anne Taylor is spearheading the effort to conduct such a study, but funding remains elusive.

The last chapter of the BiDil for heart failure saga is yet to be written.

CHAPTER XV
Treatment and Prevention of Heart Disease

It has been over a half century since my experience with Sam Farber, the patient who stimulated my quest for answers. Thanks to basic and clinical research in a number of centers, including our own, clinical practice has changed dramatically over the years. Many of the questions that confounded me in 1956 can now be effectively addressed.

Sam's terminal episode of heart failure and shock was a late consequence of damage to the heart muscle from a clot obstructing blood flow in a coronary artery six months earlier. The damage to the heart muscle had initiated a process of structural remodeling of the pumping chamber of the heart—the left ventricle—which resulted in enlargement of the chamber and a reduction of its pumping ability. This pump failure was aggravated by activation of hormone systems that constricted the arteries and placed an impedance burden on his left ventricle. He was given drugs that worsened his condition and that we now no longer use. We now know that vasodilator drugs to reduce impedance could have stabilized his pump failure and allowed his heart to begin recovering. Had drug therapy failed, he would today be placed on temporary support with a mechanical pump to supply blood flow to his body while the heart was rested.

The unwanted remodeling of the left ventricle is a silent process that we now better understand, can monitor, and can usually prevent. Opening the blocked coronary artery with urgent angioplasty has reduced damage to the heart and prevented remodeling in some. Sam certainly would have been rushed to the catheterization laboratory for angioplasty had he first appeared in the emergency room today rather than in July 1956. The problem of remodeling still exists, however, when damage is extensive. The process can be inhibited by drugs that block harmful hormone systems and by drugs that stimulate nitric oxide. Sam now would have been placed on these drugs to inhibit the remodeling, and his subsequent deterioration probably could have been prevented even if angioplasty had been delayed.

Sam Farber had long-standing hypertension that was inadequately treated in those days. Elevated blood pressure is not only a marker for structural changes in the arteries, but it also accelerates the atherosclerotic disease of the artery wall that led to his heart attack. His cholesterol levels may have been high, and this would have contributed to the atherosclerotic process in his coronary arteries. Sam's hypertension also placed a burden on his left ventricle by increasing the impedance to left ventricular ejection. This burden thickened the wall of his heart and probably contributed to the functional decline he later experienced as a consequence of structural remodeling of his left ventricle. Today's drug therapy to control blood pressure and cholesterol could have slowed the progression of his disease. Likely it would have prevented or at least greatly delayed the myocardial infarction that eventually killed him.

A dramatic change in treatment

Management in today's health care system has dramatically changed.

In 2004, nearly 50 years after Sam Farber's first hospital admission, when I was serving in my last assignment as attending physician on the University of Minnesota Hospital's cardiology service, I met Steven Fairchild, a 64-year-old lawyer brought in by ambulance from his office because of crushing chest pain. He had been whisked from the emergency room to the catheterization laboratory where a clot was found at the origin of the left anterior descending coronary artery, the large vessel that supplies the front wall of the heart. The artery was opened with a balloon catheter (angioplasty) and a stent (a plastic tube) was placed to prevent subsequent closure.

When I first saw Steven he was free of pain and talking to his office on his cell phone. His electrocardiogram showed changes of a resolving acute myocardial infarction and his echocardiogram, already performed, showed decreased contraction of the anterior wall of his left ventricle, the area of infarction. I initiated therapy with two drugs—a beta blocker, and an angiotensin converting enzyme (ACE) inhibitor—that we now know can inhibit the remodeling process and prolong life. He was also started on a statin drug to lower his cholesterol. and an anticlotting medication that we know can help prevent subsequent infarctions. He went home on day three to be fully ambulatory, and he returned to work the next week.

There is, however, a downside to this new technological management of acute MI. I hardly got to know Mr. Fairchild. The intern and resident on my service admitted 10 other patients on the day he came in. They didn't meet him until after his heart catheterization. "Door-to-balloon time"—that is, how long it takes to get the coronary artery opened—is now the standard test of hospital efficiency in managing acute myocardial infarction. I met his wife at the bedside only briefly, trying to give the two of them some insight into the nature of his disease and its management. I would probably not recognize them if I saw them on the street. We formed no doctor-patient relationship. I learned nothing of his personal life, his anxieties, his pleasures. But the cost of his three-day hospitalization far surpassed that of Sam's long hospitalization with my daily ministrations. Mr. Fairchild may come back, but it will likely be for recurrence of his coronary obstruction, not for enlargement of his ventricle. The combination of restoring blood flow to the muscle by angioplasty and the drug therapy is likely to prevent the ventricular remodeling that we have so feared in the past.

What a change in management and outcome! Is it any wonder that health care has become more expensive? How much would Steven Fairchild be willing to pay to avoid ending up like Sam Farber?

I worry, however, that the current efficiency and success in dealing with acute events like Mr. Fairchild's may lead to complacency in the effort to prevent disease. A stent in the coronary artery may even be viewed by many as a symbol of the success of our health care system.

I disagree. I think it represents a failure of the system—a failure to prevent the disease. The health care system knows the difference. Prevention is cheap, emergency treatment very expensive. Furthermore, patients like Steven Fairchild continue to cost money even after acute therapy. Drug therapy, regular monitoring, and repeated procedures to keep his stent open are standard strategies.

When Mr. Fairchild was leaving the hospital I challenged the resident doctor on the medical service. "Why are we sending him home on a beta blocker and ACE inhibitor?" I asked.

"To prevent his ventricle from remodeling," was his glib answer.

"How do you think these drugs do that?" I asked again, thinking he might have some ideas, or better still, ask me something that might elicit a dialogue about the complex mechanisms initiating cell growth and chamber enlargement. I wanted to explain to him the gaps still present in our knowledge. I wanted to express my uncertainty about the solidity of even our own observations, the possibility that continued investigation may uncover a new cellular mechanism that we have not explored.

"I guess I don't know," the resident doctor answered. His body language suggested he didn't much care.

"When do you think we learned about this?" I persisted, hoping he might identify some of the published work by our center and others.

He shrugged, glancing impatiently at the stack of charts of patients awaiting discharge. (This was just prior to the adoption of electronic records in our hospital and the replacement of paper with an electronic keypad). He was obviously intolerant of an old professor's outdated pedagogical style.

I released him back to his work.

It's published now, I thought, and this doctor thinks it's known. He's not much interested in the process of discovery or the unknown. He'll change his views if needed when new publications become available. For now he has work to do and he's comfortable knowing the right thing to do. It's certainly a less stressful way to survive as an overworked physician in a complicated, technologically advanced environment. But it emphasizes a shift in our profession. When diagnostic and therapeutic tools were limited we had time to think and reason about mechanisms of disease that we were incapable of treating. Now we have so many tools at our disposal that many physicians spend their time *doing* rather than *thinking*. In that environment, the challenge and excitement of discovery has been replaced by a dedication to efficiency.

But there is so much we still don't know. I worry that frenetic application of our current tools will inhibit the creative process on which new knowledge depends.

Challenging tradition

In every generation there have been those who challenge conventional wisdom by seeking new insights into problems that seem not to be resolved. It is they who will continue us on the path to understanding cardiovascular disease so that future generations can be more effectively freed of its complications.

If medicine is to fulfill its mission of improving the health of the people, it must shift its emphasis from treating disease to preventing disease. An ancient Chinese philosopher once claimed that average physicians treat end-stage disease, good physicians treat advancing disease and great physicians prevent disease. What we were doing with Steve Fairchild, and had failed to do with Sam Farber, was to prevent disease from progressing. This is a critical strategy when disease already has advanced to the stage of illness. But the higher goal for medicine would be to prevent the symptomatic disease from developing in the first place. In the case of cardiovascular disease, that would greatly reduce health care costs and profoundly prolong healthy life.

Could Sam Farber's or Steve Fairchild's myocardial infarctions have been prevented? Studies over the last 20 years have documented the effectiveness of drugs in slowing progression of vascular and cardiac disease. If started early enough in individuals with cardiovascular abnormalities likely to progress, I am confident that myocardial infarctions and other cardiovascular morbid events can be prevented, or at least delayed until people have lived a full life. Since heart attacks, strokes and other cardiovascular events currently account for more than half the deaths in the Western world, the future could be very different from the present.

But many questions remained unanswered. How can we identify individuals in need of such drug therapy? How much of Sam's and Steve's disease was a consequence of their genes and how much of their environment? Why do some people suffer at a young age and others live past 100 without morbid events? Are there important individual variables that determine illness risk? Can these individual variables be predicted from study of the human genome, or should we focus instead on phenotypes, those markers of the disease process and the body's response to that process? Can we define the presence of early disease by simple non-invasive measurements of cardiac and vascular function and structure? How early in life can we find the tell-tale signs that can predict the likelihood of future trouble? When should we consider intervening to possibly alter the progression of early abnormalities likely to progress to symptomatic disease? What is the best way to intervene?

The transition to prevention

These questions were all in my mind when I decided in the mid-1990s to shift my research emphasis from the treatment of heart failure to the prevention of cardiovascular disease. This decision led to the development in 2000 of the Rasmussen Center for Cardiovascular Disease Prevention and the recruitment of new colleagues dedicated to preventing disease. With the help of Dr. Daniel Duprez from Belgium, Natalia Florea from Moldova and Lynn Hoke from Iowa, we have undertaken innovative studies that may change the way we detect and treat early disease. Our long-term goal is ambitious: To prevent all cardiovascular morbid events until after the age of 100.

Why did I shift my interest when I was past 65, an age when many people retire? By the mid-1990s academic medicine and the specialty of cardiology were changing. New therapy had become standard practice to improve symptoms and survival in heart failure. The catheterization laboratory was becoming a management site more than a diagnostic laboratory, with an emphasis on procedures to open arteries and on devices to control rhythm abnormalities. The focus was less on discovery than on effective delivery of contemporary management. Hospitals and universities were recruiting for cardiologists with an interest in heart failure to help build their clinical programs.

I had organized in the early 1990s a society, the Heart Failure Society of America (HFSA), and served as its first President. My uniquely talented, long-term departmental administrator at the University, Cheryl Yano, after assisting in administering the business of the Society as part of her University duties, became its full-time Executive Director in new office space. The Society now numbers about 1500 clinicians, scientists, nurses and allied health care workers who are enthusiastically improving management of heart failure.

I also started the first medical journal devoted to research in heart failure, the *Journal of Cardiac Failure*, and served as its first editor-in-chief. It is now one of the leading cardiovascular journals, now edited by Gary Francis, and is an integral part of the HFSA. It was clear that I was no longer needed to stimulate the field.

The Cardiovascular Division was stable with outstanding senior leadership. I had asked Gary Francis, who was overseeing research at the V.A., to come to the University Hospital to direct our acute cardiac care program. To replace Gary at the V.A. I was fortunate to recruit a highly skilled and senior investigative cardiologist from India. Inder Anand, a Sikh and former Rhodes scholar with a remarkable background of research accomplishment in England and India, was ready to escape from his politically unstable country. He assumed his new position with enthusiasm and brought to it superb judgment and energy. It was Inder who became a close collaborator and key contributor to our heart failure studies of valsartan in Val-HeFT and BiDil in A-HeFT. We now had experts overseeing all the clinical and research areas of cardiology.

Changes in the clinical demands on cardiologists were accompanied by changes in academic medicine as a whole. Research, education and scholarship were being replaced by bottom-line economics. Academic medical programs had to generate income to be viable. Cardiology was a potential cash cow for departments of medicine because of the lucrative nature of many of the procedures that cardiologists performed. Revenue became the driving force of our cardiology program, and I was ill-suited for the mission. In 1996 I resigned as Director of the Division after 22 years in the position.

I was prepared to change my focus. Heart failure and acute myocardial infarction were now being treated by highly trained specialists with unique skills, many of them graduates of our program. Even though there was much more to learn, management had improved so much that mortality rates had greatly declined. I was troubled, however, by the continuing occurrence of these morbid events that I thought we should be able to prevent. Why wait for people to develop advanced disease, like myocardial infarction and heart failure, that needs aggressive and expensive therapy, if we could have prevented the progression of asymptomatic disease had we known it existed? Few if any were pursuing this important area of research. It was a vacuum that drew me in, as it always did.

In resigning as Division Head I made a deal with the dean and departmental chairman. I would remain active on the faculty if they would support me to initiate an innovative prevention program aimed at identifying and treating early cardiovascular disease that had not yet become symptomatic. I was convinced that insights we had gained from mechanisms and treatment to slow progression of advanced disease could be applied earlier if we could detect asymptomatic disease likely to progress.

Arterial stiffness

What made me so confident that we could detect such early disease? For that we need to return to two topics that we introduced earlier: Nitric oxide and the CV Profilor. The CV Profilor is the instrument that we had developed years before and was discussed earlier. It analyzes the pressure waveform detected by a device placed over the pulse at the wrist and it separately calculates stiffness or elasticity of the small and large arteries. Nitric oxide is the magical gas that is generated normally in the body as well as in response to BiDil treatment, and protects the heart from structural remodeling, as described earlier.

Although nitric oxide does protect the heart from structural changes, its primary role in the body probably is to protect the arteries. The gas is released from endothelial cells, the single layer of cells that forms the inner lining of all the arteries in the body, both small and large. When endothelial cells are functioning normally they provide a constant supply of nitric oxide that bathes the artery wall and protects it from structural changes, from invasion of substances such as cholesterol and from clots that might otherwise block the lumen or channel of the artery. Endothelial dysfunction, the state when these cells no longer provide an adequate supply of nitric oxide, appears now to be a prerequisite for the development of atherosclerosis and vascular changes that lead to heart attacks and strokes. Endothelial function is fragile and may be adversely affected by smoking, obesity, a sedentary lifestyle, diabetes, hypertension and other conditions associated with atherosclerosis. Endothelial function declines with age, which increases the susceptibility to atherosclerosis.

The discovery of nitric oxide

The discovery of a chemical released by the endothelium is attributed to Bob Furchgott, a physiologist from New York who served with me on the NitroMed Scientific Advisory Board. Bob had carried out a very simple laboratory experiment. He was accustomed to studying the tone or constrictor state of isolated arteries harvested from animals that he had rigged up with measurement devices in a bathing solution. Acetylcholine is normally released by nerve endings in the body. When Bob placed acetylcholine into the bathing solution of casually collected arteries, the arteries constricted. However, when he took great care to collect them delicately, the arteries dilated. He then gently scraped way the inner lining of these arteries and found that they once again constricted. It was clear that the inner lining was responding to the acetylcholine by releasing a vasodilator substance. That substance turned out to be nitric oxide. The observation was awarded a share of the Nobel Prize in 1998.

I had been about 30 years ahead of Bob Furchgott but didn't know enough to appreciate what I had discovered. In 1960, when I arrived in Washington for my fellowship with Ed Freis, I was interested in studying the effects of sympathetic nervous system hormones on blood vessels. Rather than isolated arteries, which Furchgott chose to study, I decided to study normally functioning arteries in the human body. Patients in the V.A. Hospital often spent weeks in the hospital for relatively mild illnesses, sometimes because they had no one to care for them and nowhere to go. They were delighted to break the boredom by volunteering to be study patients, even if it involved a few needles and a few drugs.

The simplest blood vessels to study were those in the forearm, which are easy to access. All the blood flow to the arm comes from a single artery, the brachial artery, which runs from the shoulder to the elbow. Its pulsation can be felt just above the elbow crease. If one could measure blood flow into the forearm, one could inject various substances into the brachial artery to detect their effects on the downstream forearm arteries.

The method I chose to measure flow had been developed in England and involved monitoring the girth of the forearm. If the veins draining the forearm are blocked, blood flow entering the forearm will increase its volume or girth. Venous outflow can easily be blocked by a cuff on the upper arm pressured to impede the veins but not to impede arterial inflow. The only thing acutely increasing the size of the arm in this circumstance would be the rate of blood flow into the arm. If one obstructs the drainage from the arm for just 10 seconds, flow into the arm through the arteries will not be impeded and the rate of increase in arm volume becomes a measure of arterial blood inflow. Changes in forearm girth can be monitored precisely by a fine rubber tube wrapped around the forearm. In those days it was filled with mercury. As the rubber was stretched, the mercury column was narrowed and its electrical resistance would rise. We were able to monitor the resistance in the mercury column and determine precisely the rate at which the arm volume increased. That was the rate of blood flow.

My goal was to inject into the brachial artery various doses of sympathetic hormones, norepinephrine, epinephrine and certain stimulators of these hormones, to determine the magnitude of flow reduction. I had hoped variation in response to these drugs might help explain hypertension. The problem was that when I injected these drugs, expecting to see a decline in blood flow, there was often an initial and transient increase in flow. This was a mystery to me. I looked at what literature I could find from previous experiments. No one had reported such an increase. I initially thought it was a specific response to the drugs I was testing, but then I tried injecting saline or sugar water and got the same initial increase in flow.

It was clear that there was an initial vasodilator response to these injections. I tried blocking it with all the various drugs that were known to block vasodilator action, but nothing seemed to eliminate it except repeated injections. After three or four repeated injections, the vasodilator response would disappear. I spent several months pursuing this finding and finally gave up. I couldn't explain it so I felt I couldn't report it.

What I had discovered was the release of nitric oxide from the endothelium of the brachial artery in response to the mechanical stimulation of the injection. We now know that bursts of flow induce release of nitric oxide, and that the release will disappear with repeated stimuli.

Thus, the first evidence for a vasodilator release from the endothelium never was reported and my discovery lay dormant until years later, when Bob Furchgott made the observation in isolated arteries and called the substance endothelial-derived relaxing factor (EDRF). Subsequent identification of EDRF as nitric oxide released from the endothelium is what led to his sharing the Nobel Prize.

Endothelial dysfunction

Some of the subjects I studied in 1960 had a large vasodilator response and some had none at all. What we were observing, even though I didn't know it, was the variability of endothelial function. Healthy people have a vigorous response, people with endothelial dysfunction and early vascular disease have a more modest or absent response. We now know that endothelial dysfunction is a powerful predictor of who is going to develop atherosclerosis and suffer from heart attacks and strokes. Some of that variability in endothelial function may be inherited, but it can also be influenced by environmental factors such as diet and exercise.

So if you can test for endothelial dysfunction and also assess the functional and structural vascular and cardiac abnormalities that result from inadequate nitric oxide, you should be able to identify those among apparently healthy individuals who are at risk for future cardiovascular disease. That's where the CV Profilor comes in. Our early observations with this device indicated that the small arteries become stiff or inelastic in patients with early vascular disease. The stiffness appeared to develop well before other markers for disease, such as high blood pressure, became apparent. I thought it was likely the device was detecting a deficiency in nitric oxide. I set about to study it.

Nitric oxide is formed in the body from the amino acid arginine through the action of an enzyme, nitric oxide synthase. One can block the formation of nitric oxide by injecting a substituted arginine that tricks the body to act on this substance instead of arginine. Since this substituted arginine does not form nitric oxide, the body is transiently unable to synthesize nitric oxide. So injection of this so-called nitric oxide synthase inhibitor into the circulation results in transient endothelial dysfunction.

We studied the response in a group of young volunteers. The drug was available only for research and its use in man required filing an investigational new drug (IND) application to the FDA. The process is not complicated and approval not difficult. The only side-effect that had been reported to the drug was a modest rise in blood pressure that persisted only as long as the infusion was given. During the drug infusion, we monitored blood pressure and small and large artery elasticity with the CV Profilor. Invariably, the blood pressure rose slightly but stayed within normal limits. In contrast, the small arteries became very stiff. It was clear that small artery stiffness was a sensitive guide to endothelial dysfunction.

I was therefore convinced that we would be able to use simple tests that could identify individuals with endothelial dysfunction and could detect early artery or heart disease likely to progress. I thought such early detection would allow us to intervene with drugs we now knew could slow progression of this disease. The potential to eliminate heart attacks, heart failure and strokes was now closer to a reality. I thought we could change the practice of medicine.

I had a plan. I had received a sizeable donation from a philanthropic foundation operated by the Northeast State Bank in Minneapolis. For years I had taken care of the founder and Chairman of the bank, Walter Rasmussen. He had come to me with advanced cardiovascular disease that had led to myocardial infarction, heart failure and eventually a stroke. His disease progression had been slowed by the drugs I treated him with, but his decline and death were inevitable. Treatment had been instituted too late. His wife, Belva, became bank Chairman after his death. She, her family and the bank made a donation in his memory to the University of Minnesota to support my commitment to establish a center dedicated to preventing advanced cardiovascular disease. The Rasmussen Center for Cardiovascular Disease Prevention was to become my primary focus in subsequent years.

With our knowledge of the role of nitric oxide in vascular and cardiac health and our experience with inhibiting progression of disease with the therapies that we had studied, I was confident we should be able to use easily-performed tests to identify and then treat individuals with early disease likely to progress. I was dedicated to going beyond risk factors to identify the actual early disease that leads, if untreated, to heart attacks, strokes, heart failure and other lethal morbid events.

As I set out to devise the tests, I needed to establish a clinic in which the tests would be performed. I wanted an individual to interact with the patients and oversee the evaluation process. A nurse practitioner would be ideal, I thought, because they are patient-oriented, well-trained and can bill directly for patient care. I put in ad in the local paper and had a robust response from nurse practitioners who were seeking a new opportunity in health care. One applicant, a young, energetic, personable and experienced nurse practitioner from Iowa seemed ideal. She understood the goal and the process. Lynn Hoke oversaw establishment of the Rasmussen Center and has remained a key to its success over the past decade.

A series of 10 tests have now become the basis of a routine diagnostic visit to the Rasmussen Center for Cardiovascular Disease Prevention at the University of Minnesota. These tests include arterial elasticity assessment, measurement of blood pressure response to an exercise test, ultrasound visualization of the carotid artery in the neck and the left ventricle of the heart, a photograph of the retina to measure small arteries in the eye, a urine test for albumin, and an electrocardiogram and blood test for natriuretic peptide, a hormone released by the heart when it is under stress. Everyone gets a score based on the number of abnormal tests. The higher the number, the more advanced the disease. The screening is performed in one room in one hour by one technologist at a modest cost. Our technologist, Natalia Florea, has been another key to success of the program. She is unusually skilled, since she is a physician, trained as an echocardiographer in Moldova, but functioning in the U.S. as a technician because she did not seek medical training in this country.

My closest colleague in recent years has been Daniel Duprez, who I recruited from Belgium. I had originally met Daniel while I was a visiting professor in Ghent, where he was carrying out clinical research in hypertension. When academic life in Belgium was threatened by bureaucratic intervention, Daniel sought what appeared to be a more protective environment in the United States. Daniel shares my passion for preventing cardiovascular disease and has been my partner as Associate Director of the Rasmussen Center.

The Rasmussen Center

The traditional approach to prevention has been to evaluate and treat risk factors, not to identify the presence of early disease that needs treatment to slow its progression. The traditionalists are right that the higher the level of the risk factor (for example, blood pressure and cholesterol), the greater the risk for a heart attack or stroke. And they are right that drugs that reduce blood pressure and cholesterol can reduce that risk. But they are wrong that some arbitrary level of the risk factor separates those at risk from those not at risk. The presence or absence of early disease in the arteries or heart does just that. No disease, no risk. Advancing disease, high risk.

By evaluating the health of the arteries and heart by non-invasive testing that takes only an hour, we have been able to separate patients at risk from those not at risk. In those who we find to have early disease that places them at risk, blood pressure and cholesterol levels are usually below the thresholds that have been recommended for treatment. These are the individuals who in today's health care system and are being hospitalized for heart attacks, strokes or other complications of cardiovascular disease and have not been treated to reduce their risk. The dedication to risk factor thresholds for management is missing the majority of individuals at risk.

The community-wide effort to reduce risk factors by diet, weight loss, exercise and other lifestyle changes is well justified. These efforts are harmful for nobody and beneficial for everyone at risk. A reduction in risk factor levels in the community should reduce overall community risk, reduce health care costs and improve the health and well-being of the community.

But doctors treat individuals, not populations. The recommendation that health care providers focus on treating individuals with risk factors above an arbitrary level is misguided. For care givers to be asked to make therapeutic decisions on individual patients based on modest elevations of blood pressure or cholesterol is a flawed strategy. The level of these risk factor may alter their risk by 10-15%. Does that very modest discrimination justify making a therapeutic decision to treat or not to treat? This strategy results in many patients who need treatment not being treated, and others being treated when they do not need treatment.

Application of the current risk factor model to patient care is therefore inadequate. Physicians are asked to treat these risk factors—blood pressure, cholesterol, blood sugar-- only when the levels exceed a certain value. It is true that those high levels are associated with a higher risk that might justify therapy, but the problem is that the relationship between morbid events and the risk factors is a continuum, from very low to very high levels. In fact, because there are more people with risk factors below than above the threshold for treatment, most heart attacks and strokes occur in people with what is viewed as normal levels of blood pressure and cholesterol.

We have now screened over 2000 apparently healthy individuals in our center. Most have come in because they were concerned—often because of a family history—that they might be at risk for a heart attack or stroke. Two-thirds of them have had abnormalities of the function and structure of the arteries or heart that are likely to progress if untreated. All of the subsequent morbid events detected in our screened patients have occurred in patients in whom we detected such abnormalities. In the absence of these detected abnormalities, no one has suffered from a cardiac or vascular problem in the subsequent six years. Neither their blood pressure nor their cholesterol discriminated between the groups. As might be expected, healthy endothelium and arteries appear to protect people from vascular events. The success of this program at the University in identifying and treating early disease has led to another venture, an effort to establish identical centers across the country dedicated to early detection and treatment of vascular and cardiac abnormalities likely to progress in asymptomatic individuals.

The failure of risk factors to discriminate

Our data have therefore solidified my skepticism about the use of risk factor thresholds to identify and treat patients to prevent cardiovascular morbid events. We find about one-third of the population to be free of disease and therefore highly unlikely to suffer a morbid event whatever their office blood pressure, cholesterol level, diet or life-style behavior. These people shouldn't be burdened with efforts to alter their risk factors, especially if subsequent interval screening over the years demonstrates continuing artery and heart health.

Another one-third of the population has evidence for advancing disease of the arteries or heart, probably largely due to inherited traits. Whatever their blood pressure, cholesterol levels or life-style, they need treatment to protect their cardiovascular system from disease progression.

In the final third of the population we have been able to identify early disease likely to progress. Here, life-style interventions including diet and exercise are appropriate, but if these are not adequate to slow progression, intervention with drugs to protect the arteries and heart should be employed. These drugs may lower blood pressure and cholesterol levels, but their goal is to improve vascular and cardiac health. The level of the risk factor does not necessarily identify who should be treated nor the target of the therapy.

What treatments do we utilize in these otherwise healthy people with early disease? Life style changes are the most obvious, and it is far easier to motivate an individual to change his or her behavior in order to treat demonstrable disease than to modify statistically associated risk factors. Weight loss for the obese and exercise for the sedentary is obvious. Other dietary interventions can be individualized, such as consumption of fish oil and antioxidants, which are known to improve endothelial function, as do a number of drugs that can prevent morbid events and prolong life. Statins that lower cholesterol and ACE inhibitors, angiotensin receptor blockers and calcium antagonists that lower blood pressure, all can contribute to restoration of nitric oxide activity.

Similar to most efforts that challenge conventional wisdom, this approach to prevention has faced an uphill battle with traditional forces. As James W. Black, the Nobel Prize winning biochemist, wrote in his autobiography, "entrenched attitudes can absorb reformist efforts like a punching bag". It has been a challenge to convince the entrenched establishment that blood pressure and cholesterol levels—the measurements they rely on—are not the disease, but that the disease we want to treat is in the arteries and heart. Heart attacks and strokes do not occur unless there is underlying advanced disease. If this disease can be identified before it becomes symptomatic, then treatment might be remarkably effective. We still need to prove that, especially to the skeptical establishment.

Cost-effectiveness

Because of the cost of screening to the health care system, some have criticized the idea of screening to identify those in need of treatment. The cost actually is quite modest, and pales in comparison to the cost of other so-called societal preventive efforts. Airbags are an obligatory purchase with every car we buy. If one divides the cost of airbag installation by the number of lives saved annually by airbag inflation as reported by the national traffic safety bureau, as a society we are paying $25 million per life saved. We can't restrict airbag use to cars likely to be involved in an accident, but we can focus preventive lifestyle and drug therapy on those at risk.

In the current era of financial rewards to doctors, clinics, hospitals and industry for treating advanced disease, screening to prevent disease often draws yawns. It has not been in the interest of the current health care-industrial complex. The new health care reform legislation is a major step in the right direction. By emphasizing prevention and beginning the process of finding a more equitable health care reimbursement strategy, early detection and treatment may yet become an attractive economic as well as medical strategy. Even the health care reform effort, however, has underestimated the value of prevention. Calculations of future health care costs do not adequately consider the potential magnitude of benefit of preventive strategies. If we could reduce by 50-75% the incidence of morbid events like myocardial infarction, the health care savings would dwarf whatever costs the diagnostic testing and treatment would require.

I am mystified by the contrast in the medical profession's approach to cancer and heart disease. The aggressive strategy to prevent death and disability from cancer has been to screen for early disease. Doctors strongly encourage, and health insurance pays for mammograms, prostate antigen (PSA) measurement and colonoscopy. When health authorities recently recommended decreasing the frequency of mammograms because of lack of evidence for cost-effectiveness, the profession and women's groups responded angrily. Screening for early cancer is viewed as a right that should not be abrogated. Then why not cardiovascular disease?

Medicare does not routinely cover screening for cardiovascular disease in the absence of symptoms. But cardiovascular disease disables and kills far more people every year than cancer does. Early disease can be detected. Treatment for such early disease is not destructive, as it may be with cancer that requires surgical intervention or chemotherapy. Perhaps, like other aspects of health care, it's all about money. Radiologists, gastroenterologists, urologists and surgeons all generate considerable income from cancer screening. Cardiologists depend on advanced disease.

I will continue to fight for acceptance of the virtue of early detection. I envision a world free from cardiovascular morbid events during the first century of life. Sam Farber's cardiac disease could not only have been better diagnosed and far better treated, but it could have been prevented.

It all comes together

In April 2012 I was honored with a career award from the Cardio-vascular Division of the University of Minnesota, the program I had overseen for 26 years before my resignation as chief in 1996. The award was presented to me at a gala downtown event designed to trumpet the accomplishments of the program to an assemblage of community leaders and potential donors. I was not made aware of the honor until after Syma and I had arrived in our formal attire. I was notified that a program planner would escort me after dinner to the front of the ballroom where I was to stand in the stage wing as the presenter summarized my accomplishments, and then to walk across the stage and accept the plaque.

I am always uncomfortable in those settings. The litany of my accomplishments always seems to both belittle and inflate what I did. It may suggest to the audience that the plaque is a suitable award for my research, that commendation is what may have driven me. Why do we pursue such difficult challenges? Is it the desire to help mankind? Is it the desire to leave our mark on the world? Or is it the search for answers to burning questions? It may be the insatiable desire to understand what we are doing and why we are doing it. It may be the fervent hope that the Sam Farbers of the world do not face a bleak future because of the ignorance of our health care providers.

I had consumed several glasses of wine by the time my escort arrived at the table. I was a bit unsteady on my feet. By the time I arrived in the privacy of the stage wing to await my entrance I drifted into a dream-like state in which I saw an image. It wasn't of my parents, who provided the genes and environment to set me on my path. It wasn't of Syma and my children and grandchildren, who I love and who have supported me every step of the way. It wasn't of my colleagues, whose intellectual and physical collaboration have been critical to everything I accomplished. It was an image that at first I didn't recognize until I focused on the commanding figure and the dark hair pulled back off her face.

It was Naomi Farber. She was smiling.

GLOSSARY

ACE (angiotensin converting enzyme) inhibitor
> A drug that blocks the formation of the blood vessel constricting hormone, angiotensin.

Acute myocardial infarction (AMI)
> Damage and subsequent scarring of a region of the heart muscle because of interruption of blood flow as a result of a clot causing obstruction in a coronary artery.

Alpha receptors
> A site on the wall of blood vessels that induces constriction of the artery or vein when stimulated by certain hormones, especially norepinephrine.

Amlodipine
> A drug that relaxes arteries by inhibiting the cellular action of calcium; a calcium antagonist.

Angiotensin
> A potent arterial constrictor formed by the action on a blood protein of renin coming from the kidney.

Angiotensin receptor blocker
> A drug that blocks the action of angiotensin by interfering with the angiotensin receptor on blood vessels and the heart.

Atherosclerosis

> A disease process in the wall of arteries that thickens the wall and results in plaques containing fatty material on their inner lining.

Autoregulation

> A poorly understood physiologic process in which the heart or arteries alter their function in response to a perceived pressure or flow change.

Beta blockers

> Drugs which interfere with the beta receptor's ability to respond to norepinephrine.

Beta receptor

> A site in proximity to nerve endings in the heart that responds to a hormone, especially norepinephrine, by increasing the force and rate of the heart's contraction.

Bioassay

> Measurement of the potency of a drug or chemical by its action on a living tissue or animal

Blood pressure

> The pressure within the arterial system generated by the pumping of the left ventricle of the heart; systolic is when the left ventricle is emptying, diastolic is between beats.

Brachial artery

> The artery that runs from the shoulder to the elbow and provides all the blood flow to the forearm.

Capillary

> The terminal end of the arterial system where the arterial blood nourishes the tissues, from which it is recollected in veins to return to the heart.

Captopril

The first oral angiotensin receptor inhibitor (ACE inhibitor) developed for the treatment of hypertension.

Cardiac arrest

Cessation of the heart's contraction, usually because of the failure of the electrical signal to beat.

Cardiac output

The amount of blood pumped by the heart in a given interval, usually measured in liters per minute.

Carvedilol

A sympathetic nervous system inhibitor that blocks the stimulating effect of norepinephrine on the beta receptors of the heart. It also inhibits other hormonal systems that contribute to its effect on the heart and blood vessels.

Cirrhosis

A disease of the liver characterized by scarring and impaired liver function. Excess alcoholic intake is a common cause.

Compliance

The stiffness of a material, measured as the pressure required to stretch or deform it.

Constriction

The process by which the smooth muscle in the wall of a blood vessel is stimulated to reduce the caliber of the lumen and its column of blood.

Coronary artery

The blood vessels that run on the outside of the heart and nourish the heart's muscle or myocardium.

Constriction

> A state of the arteries in which smooth muscle contraction reduces the size of the artery's lumen or blood channel.

Data safety and monitoring board (DSMB)

> An expert committee selected to oversee the conduct of a clinical trial. Members are not to have any involvement in the conduct of the study.

Defibrillator

> A device that delivers an electrical shock to the heart in order to terminate a chaotic and life-threatening heart beat disorder.

Diastole

> The period of the cardiac cycle during which the heart is relaxed and fills with blood in anticipation of the next beat.

Digoxin or digitalis

> Drugs derived from the digitalis plant and used to increase the force of contraction of heart muscle.

Dilation

> A state of relaxation of the smooth muscle in an artery that increases the size of the lumen.

Diuretics

> Drugs that increase the flow of urine by an action on the kidney to increase salt excretion.

Dose-response curve

> Data collected at escalating doses of a drug to identify the relationship between a given dose and the desired effect of the drug.

Ejection fraction

> A measure of the function of the heart defined as the fraction of blood in the heart at the end of the filling phase (diastole) that is ejected during contraction.

Enalapril
> An angiotensin converting enzyme inhibitor used to treat hypertension and heart failure.

Endothelium
> The inner lining of all arteries that is the source of nitric oxide release as well as that of other substances that influence the tone and structure of the artery wall.

Felodipine
> A calcium antagonist used to treat hypertension and the drug tested in V-HeFT III.

Flosequinon
> A vasodilator drug that was demonstrated not to have a favorable effect on the course of heart failure.

Genotype
> The pattern of DNA in a given individual.

Heart failure
> A common clinical condition in which abnormalities of the left ventricle's contraction or filling leads to impaired heart function and to symptoms such as fatigue, shortness of breath and leg swelling.

Hormones
> Chemical substances released into the circulation from the tissues of an organ and exerting their effect remotely on other organs.

Hydralazine
> A vasodilator drug traditionally used to treat hypertension but now advocated for the treatment of heart failure in combination with isosorbide dinitrate in some patients with heart failure.

Hypertension

A common clinical condition currently defined by a resting blood pressure higher than 149/90 mmHg.

Hypertrophy

A state of cellular enlargement usually used in reference to structural enlargement of the left ventricle of the heart.

Impedance

The forces opposing the ejection of blood from the heart into the arterial system.

Inotropism

The property of increasing the force of the heart muscle's contraction.

Ischemia

A state in which an organ or tissue is deprived of adequate blood flow for its nutrition.

Isosorbide dinitrate

An orally active drug in the nitrate family that exerts its effect to relax arteries on release of nitric oxide

Left ventricle

The pumping chamber of the heart.

Left ventricular filling pressure

The pressure of the blood filling the left ventricle before its next contraction.

Levophed

The commercial preparation of norepinephrine used to induce arterial wall constriction.

Morbid events
> Clinical conditions that produce symptoms that impair the health and quality of life of individuals

Myocardium
> The heart muscle, which is composed of both myocytes and cellular and tissue elements that hold the myocytes together.

Myocyte
> The contracting cell that makes up the bulk of the heart's left ventricle

Natriuretic peptides
> Substances released by the heart that stimulate the kidney to increase its elimination of salt from the body.

Nitrate
> A generic term for drugs that exert their effect by releasing nitric oxide.

Nitric oxide (NO)
> A gas normally released from the inner lining of the arteries and from the inner lining of the heart and preserves the health of the arteries and heart.

Nitroglycerin
> A nitrate drug that is absorbed from under the tongue and is effective in generating nitric oxide to relax arteries.

Nitroprusside
> An intravenous drug that releases nitric oxide and is effective in acutely lowering blood pressure and in improving the function of the failing left ventricle.

NO
> The abbreviation for nitric oxide.

Norepinephrine

> The hormone released by the sympathetic nervous system that has powerful effects on the blood vessels and the heart.

P-value

> A statistical term based on a calculation to assess the likelihood that an observation is valid rather than a play of chance.

Perfusion

> The blood flow to an organ.

Phenotype

> The physiological state of an individual determined from a study of function and structure.

Placebo

> A dummy medication made to look like a real medication used in a blinded clinical trial.

Plaques

> Accumulations of cholesterol, often accompanied by calcium, that form on the inner lining of arteries and represents the atherosclerotic process.

Prazosin

> A drug that inhibits the constrictor effect of norepinephrine on blood vessels through blockade of the alpha receptors in the vessel wall.

Radial artery

> The artery at the wrist that is used for taking an individual's pulse and for placement of a device to record the arterial waveform.

Randomization

> The requirement in a clinical trial to enter eligible patients by a system that will lead to similar characteristics in those given one therapy versus other therapies.

Resistance

The opposition to blood flow induced primarily by the small arteries, the narrowing of which obligates the heart to generate a higher pressure to maintain blood flow.

Remodeling

The structural changes in the heart and blood vessels that may lead to adverse consequences.

Renin

A hormone, released by the kidney especially in response to a fall in blood pressure, that facilitates the production of angiotensin, a potent substance that constricts arteries and raises blood pressure.

Right ventricle

The heart chamber that receives blood from the veins and pumps it to the lungs.

Sarcomeres

The basic units of heart muscle cells that contribute to the cellular contraction.

Shock

A circulatory state when blood flow is inadequate to nourish the organs of the body.

Stent

A plastic sleeve that can be placed, through a catheter, into an obstructed artery to keep the artery open.

Stroke volume

The amount of blood pumped from the heart with each beat.

Sympathetic nervous system

The nerve pathways originating in the brain and spinal column that respond to stress with activation of blood vessel constriction and heart stimulation.

Systole

That portion of the cardiac cycle when the heart is contracting.

Thrombosis

A clot of blood in an artery or vein that obstructs the blood flow.

V-HeFT

A series of clinical trials, Vasodilator Heart Failure Trials, that evaluated the effectiveness of drugs that relaxed the artery on mortality and morbidity.

Valsartan

A drug that blocks the action of angiotensin on the blood vessels and heart and is used to treat hypertension and heart failure.

Vasoconstriction

The state in which the arteries are constricted in an effort to raise blood pressure.

Vasodilators

Drugs that relax the arteries to reduce the resistance against which the heart is ejecting blood.

Vasopressin

A hormone released by the pituitary gland that constricts blood vessels and stimulates the kidneys to conserve water in the body.

Vesnarinone

A drug that increases the force of cardiac contraction. In a clinical trial it had an adverse effect on survival in patients with severe heart failure.

About the Author

Jay Cohn, M.D., is Professor of Medicine at the University of Minnesota Medical School and Director of the Rasmussen Center for Cardiovascular Disease Prevention. He was Director of the University's Cardiovascular Division from 1974-96. He is widely recognized for his contributions to an understanding of hypertension, coronary artery disease, myocardial infarction and heart failure. He is the author of over 750 scientific papers and has been honored by the American Heart Association, American College of Cardiology, American College of Physicians, American Society of Hypertension, Heart Failure Society of America, American Association for the Advancement of Science, Cornell University and the University of Minnesota for his research accomplishments. He has served as president of four national and international societies and is co-editor of a major textbook, Cardiovascular Medicine. He holds a number of patents on devices and drugs used to diagnose and treat cardiovascular disease. While continuing to pursue his clinical and research efforts at the University of Minnesota, he and his wife, Syma, now spend the winter months on Longboat Key, Florida, where golf and tennis blend with the arts life of Sarasota.

34024589R10172

Made in the USA
Charleston, SC
25 September 2014